Caring for Equality

The African American History Series

This series takes both chronological and thematic approaches to topics and individuals crucial to an understanding of the African American experience. The books in this series, in lively prose by established scholars, are aimed primarily at nonspecialists. They focus on topics in African American history that have broad significance and place them in their historical context. While presenting sophisticated interpretations based on primary sources and the latest scholarship, the authors tell their stories in a succinct manner, avoiding jargon and obscure language. They include selected documents that allow readers to judge the evidence for themselves and to evaluate the authors' conclusions. Bridging the gap between popular and academic history, these books will bring the African American story to life.

Current Titles in the Series

Caring for Equality

A History of African American Health and Healthcare

David McBride

ROWMAN & LITTLEFIELD
Lanham • Boulder • New York • London

Published by Rowman & Littlefield
A wholly owned subsidiary of The Rowman & Littlefield Publishing Group, Inc.
4501 Forbes Boulevard, Suite 200, Lanham, Maryland 20706
www.rowman.com

Unit A, Whitacre Mews, 26-34 Stannary Street, London SE11 4AB, United Kingdom

British Library Cataloguing in Publication Information Available

Library of Congress Cataloging-in-Publication Data

Names: McBride, David, author.
Title: Caring for equality : a history of African American health and
    healthcare / David McBride.
Description: Lanham : Rowman & Littlefield, [2018] | Series: African American
    history series | Includes bibliographical references.
Identifiers: LCCN 2018008806 (print) | LCCN 2018009169 (ebook) | ISBN
    9781442260603 (Electronic) | ISBN 9781442260597 (cloth : alk. paper)
Subjects: | MESH: Minority Health--history | African Americans--history |
    Health Services Accessibility--history | Healthcare Disparities--history |
    Slaves--history | Racism--history | History, Modern 1601- | United States
Classification: LCC RA448.5.N4 (ebook) | LCC RA448.5.N4 (print) | NLM WA 11
    AA1 | DDC 362.108996/073--dc23
LC record available at https://lccn.loc.gov/2018008806

♾ ™ The paper used in this publication meets the minimum requirements of American National Standard for Information Sciences Permanence of Paper for Printed Library Materials, ANSI/NISO Z39.48-1992.

Printed in the United States of America

This book is dedicated to the memories of my mother, Ruth McBride Jordan, and my older brother, William. Throughout his life as a physician, Billy taught his younger brother that good medicine is not just a science, but an art and a belief. Billy was a deeply religious fellow who would remind us all, as he no doubt did others in his life: "The steps of a good man are ordered by the Lord, and he delights in his way. Though he fall, he shall not be utterly cast down, for the Lord upholds him with his hand" (Psalm 37:23–24)

Contents

Acknowledgments

There are many who supported me throughout the many seasons I worked on this book. Sincere thanks to Jackie Moore, Nina Mjagki, Jon Sisk, and Kate Powers, editors at Rowan & Littlefield, for working with me to shape this book. Jackie in particular went well beyond the standard editor's role, providing incisive input at every step of my manuscript's development. Mary Gage, independent scholar and friend, read early portions of the manuscript, giving me valuable orientation for the later overall book. The personnel of Pattee Library at Pennsylvania State University provided untiring help with sifting through Pattee's mountains of academic materials and innumerable gateways to digital archives. It was under their expert guidance that I garnered much of the factual content of this book. Also, the bibliographic resources at the National Library of Medicine (Bethesda, Maryland) were indispensable in my research of all aspects of this book. Last, I would like to thank my longtime mentors and friends from Denison University: Ronald Santoni, Henry Durand, Monroe and Sheila Little, and Catherine "Kit" Andrews.

There is a large family and many close friends to thank for supporting me throughout the years I worked on this book. Among the family: my kids, Patrice and Julian, and their mother, Angelike Simons (sadly, now deceased), and siblings Andrew Dennis, Richard, Helen, Rosetta, Dotty, Judy, James, Hunter, Henry, and Kathy, as well as nephew William. Two new additions to this parade of inspiration are Mason and Mateo, my preschool-aged grandsons. They are in for about two decades of formal education that I hope amplifies their inherent warmth, curiosity, and happiness. On the "second line" of supporters have been in-laws Gary, Val, Eva, Rose, and kids; nephew Gyasi and niece Maya; and a host of others. Additionally, I could not have completed this book without the spirited counsel and insights of my friends Darryl Thomas; Gary King; Lorraine Brown, and her children, Dee and Kevin; Donna and Barry King; Merida and Nuria Padro; Alexine Pinder; Sheila Inge; and Roxana Gearhart.

Introduction

America in the twenty-first century has one of the most technologically advanced healthcare systems in the world. To fully understand America's rise to leadership in modern medical care, the trials and triumphs of black Americans in medical history must be told. This book provides an exploration of the black American medical and health journey. It starts in the earliest prescientific phase of American healthcare and ends with the scientific medicine of today's postindustrial and global America. It will trace the black (or African American) health and medical experience from the era of slavery to the present. The black struggle for health equality was a vital contribution to modern America's development into a global leader in healthcare delivery and medical science.

The book begins with slavery, the premodern period of U.S. medicine. Like American colonial and early Republic society as a whole, early black American healthcare centered on practical medical cures and folk healthcare. However, starting in the late nineteenth century, medicine increasingly unified around the advancing biological sciences. New fields of bacteriology, epidemiology, public health administration, and modern physiology emerged. These, in turn, gave rise to "academic"-based medicine for both the physician and the hospital in the twentieth century. Yet black doctors and other healthcare givers were kept on the margins of the new medical professions and hospital institutions.

The central thesis of *Caring for Equality* is that health progress for American blacks resulted from the steady influence of advocates and institutional forces pursuing what I call the *health equality ideal*—that is, the principle that the health of black Americans could and should be of an equal priority to that of whites and other Americans. Related to this ideal was the understanding that African Americans themselves should have access to medical education and should be able to perform medical care at the highest levels of academic and professional expertise. The central narrative of this book follows the ups and downs in the way this ideal shaped the participation of blacks in healthcare institutions, as well as how they had an impact on the health progress of black Americans. We will see that in their pursuit of the health equality ideal, blacks and their allied health activists and political supporters constantly struggled to widen black opportunities in medical fields, hospital services, and community healthcare resources.

By focusing on the black American medical and health experience, this book bears out John Hope Franklin's simple, yet prescient idea. Throughout America's past, "[t]he specter of color" has been "the unseen force that influences public policy as well as private relationships...even when it goes unmentioned."[1] By concentrating on the historic role of black Americans in medicine and their collective health during the nation's modern evolution, the reader can see the foundations of our current-day social and medical strengths and weaknesses. For American blacks, this evolution has been a story of progress, but also of persistent disparities and intermittent public crises in healthcare provision and health status.

Despite the largely discriminatory policies and practices that blacks confronted within the nation's medical institutions, as the United States took on the character of a full-fledged welfare-state nation mobilized to eliminate poverty, overall black American health improved. Furthermore, blacks built self-reliant core institutions and community life to sustain black health with or without assistance from government and dominant medical institutions. They also mobilized with progressive allies to force power holders in the medical sector to address black health inequality.

Fundamental biological, environmental, and medical resources that improved the health of blacks also raised the health levels for whites, Latino Americans, Native Americans, and other ethnic segments of the American population. However, adequate distribution of these resources depended overwhelmingly on the success or failure of black struggles within the nation's broader political and economic institutions. From the slavery era to the modern day, the self-conscious struggle by black health-rights activists, supported by progressive white and minority allies, served as a catalyst for achieving better healthcare for all working-class Americans.

Caring for Equality covers the medical care and health experience of American blacks as it unfolded in the key phases of national life, medical science, and race relations. Chapters 1 and 2 focus on the period from slavery through to the early 1900s, including the Civil War and Reconstruction periods, and what some historians have called the Nadir decades (that is, the 1880s through the 1900s), with the rise of segregation. Chapter 1 describes the ways in which enslaved and free African-Americans developed social and cultural practices, as well as indigenous and trained "doctors" and midwives. Combining these developments enabled American blacks to sustain health despite their horrific living conditions under institutionalized slavery. Chapter 2 covers the Civil War and Reconstruction eras and the decades that followed. At this time, the federal government embarked on its "first" Reconstruction to build up the health of the ex-slaves and assist in educating trained physicians and nurses. However, in the years after Reconstruction the "separate but equal" doctrine began to take root deeply within American political and public life. U.S. blacks began developing their own medical institutions and healthcare network. Leaders and white supporters from within segregated black America nurtured self-reliant black medical and nursing professions, as well as health promotion resources within community, religious, and folk institutions.

Chapter 3 examines the national network of black medical professionals during the so-called Jim Crow period. These are the decades of the Progressive Era, World War I, the Twenties, and the New Deal. With the onrush of racist Jim Crow laws and social practices nationwide, millions of blacks in the South were forced to live under the neoslavery of the sharecropping system. Still, blacks built and sustained their own self-reliant "Black Medical World." This black healthcare sector functioned effectively despite the Jim Crow segregation rampant throughout the nation's medical and public health establishment. This chapter also covers the impact of the Great Migration on black America's health predicament, and finally the New Deal federal programs that greatly improved the healthcare as well as the living conditions for the nation's blacks, especially the poor and unemployed.

Chapter 4 focuses on the impact of World War II and America's welfare-state policies in moving the health-equality ideal forward in the medical sector's engagement with black soldiers and civilians. It describes the first wave of civil rights skirmishes that questioned hospital segregation, as well as the color bar in the medical professions and organizations. Chapter 5 describes the momentous influence the civil rights movement and urban black riots had on federal and city government's commitment to black health equality from the late 1960s through the 1970s. As the Civil Rights Act of 1964 and the "War on Poverty" domestic programs took hold, the overall health of blacks, as well as their access to hospital care, medical education, and healthcare jobs, made great strides. In this so-called Second Reconstruction for black Americans, the federal government pressured hospitals, healthcare agencies, and medical profession schools in both the North and the South to more fully integrate.

Chapter 6 focuses on the late 1970s through the 1990s. Gradually the landmark federal healthcare insurance and programs of the 1960s and early 1970s proved insufficient for new impediments to black health and medical care that later arose during the 1980s and 1990s. For one, immense changes occurred in the urban social and environmental landscape in which blacks lived. In many black urban neighborhoods, new forms of concentrated poverty developed, producing "New Ghetto" conditions. In this context, a national black health crisis unfolded, especially for blacks who lacked health insurance and had little protection from poverty and crime. Health catastrophes like AIDS, tuberculosis (TB), and illicit drug use also outmatched the available healthcare resources in many black communities.

Finally, chapter 7 examines how black health leadership and communities rose to meet the challenges posed by the AIDS epidemic and the related social crises. In the period since the 1990s, the nation moved into a new conservative political climate, and experienced a shift toward neoliberal economics and domestic programming. Under neoliberal economics and conservative politics, public resources such as schools, criminal justice facilities, neighborhood development, and health insurance for the poor and elderly become market-driven and, in many cases, privatized. Fighting environmental injustice also became a major equality ideal that guided the struggle to protect and improve black community health.

In this most recent period, new crises and threats to black health emerged, many of which are environmental in origin. These include natural disasters like Hurricane Katrina and postindustrial conditions such as polluted housing and drinking water. Others involve widespread chronic diseases and behavioral problems linked to inadequate medical screening and intervention, living conditions, and family behaviors. Black Americans presently struggle to envision and advocate for health equality, as they did in earlier historical periods, but now in an even more socially globalized society. In short, the struggle by the black American citizenry for healthcare equality remains an integral part of their overall struggle for political and social equality.

Chapter One

Slavery and the Medical Roots

Africa and the New World

On a fall day in 1788, the young Republic's most prominent medical figure, Dr. Benjamin Rush, met with a Dr. James Derham. Dr. Rush had been the surgeon general for the Continental Army and was then a leading scientific and civic figure throughout the nation. Derham, a slave, born in Philadelphia, had lived under three slave masters who were doctors. One of the nation's first African American medical doctors, Derham had journeyed to his medical trade as a child of slavery.

While owned by Dr. Robert Dove of New Orleans, Derham demonstrated a natural aptitude for mastering surgical and medical maneuvers. Through his own efforts, Derham became broadly educated, as well as fluent in several languages. Allowed to purchase his freedom, Derham blossomed into a talented and trusted doctor, widely sought after among the free people of color and slave populations of bustling New Orleans. Dr. Rush came away from his discussion with Derham that day in 1788 deeply impressed. Rush later wrote: "I have conversed with him upon most of the acute and epidemic diseases of the country where he lives. . . . I expected to have suggested some new medicines to him, but he suggested many more to me."

While Dr. Derham's medical talents had exceeded the expectations of Dr. Rush, he was one of countless black Americans of high accomplishment in the medical field during the centuries of slavery, the Civil War, Jim Crow segregation, and urban poverty. But this historic drive by black Americans and their allies to improve health and medical care for themselves developed its foundation during the era of slavery and abolitionist struggle. Through strong spiritual belief, collective willpower, intellectual ingenuity, and physical and nutritional dexterity, blacks soundly refuted the doom predicted for

1

their race by the nation's white political, intellectual, and scientific elites. These white leaders argued that blacks could never be as healthy as whites or qualify as medical providers due to the alleged physical deficiencies of the black African race, coupled with the black's social demoralization as a result of slavery and segregation.

The more than two-centuries-long experience of slavery contributed to the spiritual and intellectual strength that black Americans needed for their perilous health and medical journey. Historians estimate that close to twelve million Africans were transported across the Atlantic. They provided the pivotal labor for the European colonizers of the New World. Between 1619 and 1807, about one half million Africans arrived by ship into the territory that comprises today's United States. The bulk of the enslaved Africans landed in British North America between 1720 and 1780. These generations of slaves formed the core ancestors of most of today's modern black American population. Newly enslaved Africans received healthcare from one or a combination of three sources: self-care based on their African cultural traditions; the apprentice-trained doctors or lay caregivers supplied by their individual owners; or local folk healers from the long-standing African American community itself.

No matter who rendered practical healthcare, the health of both the owners and slaves could benefit from the environmental and nutritional conditions in which they lived and worked. Some scholars emphasize the totality of the slave owners' control over enslaved people, to the point that slaves themselves even internalized their powerlessness. However, the health and healthcare aspirations of slaves and the free black populations indicate the opposite. The slave master class never fully extinguished the natural environment's positive contributions to the health of the slaves, nor the slave's own healthcare institutions, family institutions, and psychological resilience. Enslaved women from Africa had a rich cultural knowledge of natural birth control and abortifacients from their indigenous cultures. Throughout their passage into life under slavery, the women concealed this indigenous knowledge and practices from slave traders and owners. This enabled many slave women to maintain some freedom over their bodies even under the constant pressure of slave owners subjecting the female slaves to inhumane breeding practices.

Overall, the enslaved person's health was under constant peril. Harmful physical and physiological conditions such as poor diets, inadequate shelter, violence, and psychological stress were endemic to slave life. Some of these conditions triggered biological processes of specific diseases. Moreover, slaves were subject to the frequent misdiagnoses or prejudiced callousness of physicians and other health practitioners in charge of tending ill slaves.

Nutrition was a key factor in the health of all of the slaves. The slave's food supply derived from two sources. Food was provided by slave masters and operators of the particular plantation or farm on which the slave dwelled. Some slaves were able to gather foods year-round from their own personal garden plots if they were fortunate to have them; others obtained food by foraging, hunting, and fishing. The types of food and cash crops grown depended on the immediate land and natural resources surrounding the plantation or farm. In turn, the larger geographic environment and regional climate influenced the plantation's overall land conditions.

The most common staples of the slave diet were corn and pork, neither of which is particularly nutritious. Many slaves were lactose intolerant and, consequently, did not drink milk, a key source of nutrients. Slaves often had niacin deficiency, an unhealthy dietary condition that causes pellagra. This disease produces a variety of symptoms, including dermatitis, mental confusion, diarrhea, physical weakness, sensitivity to light, and heart problems. Early stages of pellagra disease also increase susceptibility to pneumonia and tuberculosis infection. However, when observing early pellagra symptoms in slaves, Southern physicians described the symptoms as the results of African racial peculiarities and often used the popular term "black tongue" disease.

Likewise, the various regional climates and crops of the plantations strongly influenced the work hazards as well as threats from local infectious diseases and epidemics that the slaves faced. In the upper South—Maryland, Virginia, and North Carolina, for instance—plantations and farms raised mainly cotton and tobacco. In areas within the lower South—Louisiana, South Carolina, Florida, Mississippi, Georgia, and Alabama—sugarcane and rice were major crops. The cultivation of these different crops created specific health problems and regional diseases. For example, slaves on rice plantations in hot, humid low-country Georgia and South Carolina worked in swamps and marshes. Building dikes, planting, and harvesting in water-soaked soil, these slaves suffered bites from vermin such as alligators and snakes, as well as mosquito-borne diseases such as malaria and yellow fever. Slaves on sugar plantations experienced equally harsh work conditions. From planting to cutting cane, the wear and tear on the bodies of these slaves was intense. Cuts, exhaustion, and high suicide rates prevailed among this slave segment. Finally, typhoid fever outbreaks riddled poorly cared for slaves on the South's cotton plantations.

Slave women faced additional health concerns through pregnancy and childbirth. Forced to work and bear children at the same time, pregnancy and childbirth were trying, if not fatal, for both the mother and infant. Pregnant and nursing slaves faced daunting conditions. These included malnutrition, hard labor, unsanitary and stressful postpartum conditions, inadequate maternity care, and prevalent infectious diseases. Overall, these handicaps led to extraordinarily high levels of maternal and infant mortality among the female slaves.

In 1808 slave importation became illegal. Consequently, slave owners placed greater emphasis on increasing the numbers of slaves through natural means. In worse cases, the atrocious practice of slave breeding, or forced conjugation, occurred. In more benevolent slave households, voluntary marriage and childbearing were encouraged. Female slaves in particular felt the brunt of inhumane physical suffering. They were pressured into forced and frequent childbearing at a horrible cost to their health and the health of their infants. Foreign women travelers to southern plantations found slave women making constant appeals for help for the pain and exhaustion they were experiencing. One such traveler to a Georgia plantation in the 1830s was shocked by the conditions facing the pregnant slave women. One woman complained of "dreadful pains in the back, and internal tumor which swells with the exertion of working in the fields . . . ," she writes. "[P]robably I think, she is ruptured," she continues, and should be in "a bed in a hospital [rather than] working all day in the fields."[1]

Pregnant slave women could feign illness to manipulate decisions and practices of slave masters in ways that allowed the women to protect and strengthen their families. On large plantations, where blacks were the majority and communal ties and values were the strongest, slave women exercised more control over their lives. Women of the rice plantations, for example, had babies at older ages, suggesting later marriages. Scholars have also discovered that these women frequently regulated sex according to harvesting seasons. No doubt plantation overseers could and did violate these preferences of slave women, but the strong social bonds among the slave women themselves also acted as a protection against the threat or reality of such persistent sexual violence.

Besides female slaves enduring pregnancies, most slaves faced other forms of physical suffering. These included food and water deprivation, painful whippings, and other types of violence inflicted by slave owners and slave drivers. When the population of imported slaves dropped steeply after 1808, slave owners were driven to a contradictory approach to the health and social welfare of their slaves. On one hand, they had to inflict sufficient physical and psychological punishment to keep slaves productive workers and, for females, fertile for birthing healthy babies. On the other hand, the punishments they meted out could and often did take the health and, indeed, even the life of the slave.

Whippings, assaults with fists and wooden rods, brandings, dog bites, and gashes from chains and iron restraints left slaves with injuries, infections, and disabilities on a horrendous scale. Slaves also suffered burns, lacerations, mutilated body parts, and bone fractures either from the actions of slave drivers or from dangerous work tasks the slaves were forced to do. Additionally, the lack of protection from extreme climates was a persistent cause for illnesses, injuries, and disease among the slaves.

Slave owners were always vigilant about not overstepping the physical breaking point of their slaves. Unproductive slaves or slaves who died unexpectedly could mean financial ruin for slave owners. Therefore, regardless of the size of the plantation or household, slave owners usually saw that the master, slave physicians, or someone from within the slave community tended to the health of slaves. On the larger plantations, owners employed professional physicians who specialized in caring for slaves. They also sometimes operated on-site infirmaries or hospitals. These facilities provided conditions for rest and recovery, if the slave patients could avoid contagion and depression. On small plantations, where an owner and his family employed only a few families of slaves, the wives of the owners often looked after the health needs of the slaves.

Indeed, a major portion of the physician's finances in the antebellum South was garnered from payments received from slave owners for the care of slaves. Plantation physician care included treatment for cholera. These doctors also provided vaccinations against smallpox to slaves and others on the plantation. Slave doctors also treated slaves having difficult deliveries or other maternity conditions. Even dental problems were treated by plantation physicians.

But enslaved people also looked to their own traditions for healthcare. Throughout the black American community, both under slavery and in post-Emancipation, religious systems of health restoration that had originated in African societies before the slave trade were transplanted with varying intensities. Historians estimate that by the end of the 1700s, about twenty thousand new slaves were imported each year into the United States. As newcomers arrived in the North American colonies, they added their own African cultural practices to American ones, forming a hybrid Afro-American culture. Sociologist W. E. B. Du Bois described the religion that the first enslaved Africans delivered to Southern plantations as "nature-worship, with profound belief in invisible surrounding influences, good and bad." This worship was conducted "through incantation and sacrifice."[2] Spirituals and ceremonial music and dance were widespread throughout the slave quarters, out of the sight of slave masters. An added Christian element evolved as the result of missionary work of black Christian ministers, mostly freed blacks, as well as from "slave missions" sponsored by the nation's larger white denominations and plantation owners. The religious impulse was so strong among the slaves, they held secret meetings for worship and celebration of God if masters did not permit such gatherings.

Religious and spiritual traditions nourished enslaved people psychologically in the face of pain and death. They also provided therapeutic influences for an array of practical folk healers and their remedies. Over the generations, folk healthcare involved indigenous healers, conjurers, and religious practitioners. As local households and communities of slaves exchanged their folk-healing memories and methods, the process of what anthropologists call medical syncretism occurred, blending different traditions. The enslaved Africans also incorporated health practices they believed useful from the European and Native American health practitioners they encountered in the larger community.

As the American-born black African population grew, a vast number of folk healers emerged from this cultural and syncretic engine, along with a small sprinkling of apprenticed-trained practitioners of professional medicine. Whether within the slave quarters, the harshest work camp conditions of the large plantations, or the free black communities of the urban South and North—black Americans pursued their physical survival without white help.

The spread of African spiritualist folkways in medicine and health took different forms throughout the various African diaspora cultures of the Western world. As a result of such imports, in North America's slave South, religion, conjure, and magic became the heart of black folk healing practices. For centuries, each slave community's individual practitioners of conjure and magic purveyed religious spiritualism and health practices throughout the slave South. In his classic *Souls of Black Folk* (1903), Du Bois described the importance of these cultural leaders of slaves, which included preachers, priests, and medicine men. They were not only the healers of the sick, but according to Du Bois, they were foundations for the post-Emancipation "Negro preacher" as well as the "Negro Church."

Conjurers, folk healers, and spiritualists were a vital thread in the social fabric of the slave communities, because they provided intimate psychological support to slaves. A former slave described the subtle blend of faith in magic, religious belief, and logic that conjurers invoked in their followers. Slaves believed these healers received their power from God, enabling them to recognize the signs that the Lord sent: "Some of the folks laugh at their beliefs and says it am [sic] superstition," according to the former slave, but actually it is the healer "knowing how the Lord reveals His laws." Indeed, in his path-breaking study, *The Slave Community: Plantation Life in the Antebellum South* (1972), John Blassingame emphasized that conjurers hold more control over slaves than even the slave masters.

Black folk healers used herbs, charms, and rituals to effect cures to ailments of all types. Conjurers and their believers called for spiritual intervention to aid with the healing of the sick, ridding someone of an enemy, or watching over a loved one. Just as white folk healers during the slave period based many of their practices on European sacred practices, likewise, conjure uses religious or metaphysical belief. However, color prejudice usually diverted white healers from empathizing with black folk spiritual and healing practices. Black folk advice and healing involving conjure frightened white slave owners and lay populations. White Christian elites saw such folk health practices—woven as they were with alien religious beliefs—as a threat to their authority. Since slaves relied on their healers, spiritualists, and religious leaders for intimate counsel and healing, these healers were inherently threatening to the authority of the slave drivers and owners. Likewise, the places and circumstances in which folk healers transmitted their knowledge were usually hidden from slave and plantation overseers and owners.

Most whites harbored disdain for conjuring. Even some black Christian ministers loathed conjurers and healers who relied on magic and spiritualism. Still, black folk healers and midwives developed abiding trust within the slave quarters. On the plantations, black healers sometimes worked alongside doctors or nurses provided by the plantation owners. Ellen Betts, an ex-slave from Texas, reported using both traditional and doctor-prescribed medicines to treat her patients, both black and white. At the same time, white medical practitioners provided by slave owners were frequently met with suspicion, if not resistance, from slaves. As for the black sections in large cities where free and slave blacks mingled, black doctors like James Derham employed their healing arts, gaining wide popularity and consistent clienteles.

Slaves passed along folk healing practices orally and through demonstration in the slave quarters, work surroundings, and places of worship. Other points of transmission for folk health remedies included public places where slaves gathered, such as markets, and the natural areas on the outskirts of the planting fields. Multigenerational households were common throughout the African American slave communities of both North and South America, and the Caribbean. These households were natural conduits for folk health values and practices. In churches, healing rituals were a common part of service. Finally, anthropologists have identified "folk clinics," which were simply any place where the folk healer routinely chose to receive "patients."

Overall, the informal health system woven together within slave communities provided channels for mental health guidance and physical healing. Through these channels, medical information was openly shared by healers with community members, who shared the same information with their neighbors. The information was then circulated once more within social institutions such as churches, communal workplaces, and the settings and clubs in which women and men participated in leisure activities. Within the formally trained medical field, medical information was usually generated and shared primarily within professional circles. By contrast, folk remedies were tested and evaluated practically. The findings were then passed along through channels wide open to all members of the slave community—whether these communities were in cities, towns, or plantation quarters. Newspapers, books, and pamphlets frequently carried information about successful folk remedies for slaves to whites living in nearby communities and towns. Articles described various illnesses and other health problems that whites presumed were unique to slaves and the possible remedies the folk healers had tried effectively or ineffectively.

Although they were suspicious of conjure practices, whites often adopted slave remedies, usually comprised of local plants, herbs, and minerals. For example, slaves used chestnut leaf tea for asthma and jimsonweed to relieve rheumatism. Sassafras root tea was supposed to have the power to "search the blood" for sickness and alleviate it. One white doctor tried milkweed or silkweed (*Asclepias syriaca*), which Virginia blacks had been using for years, as a relief for fevers and agues. He found it almost as effective as quinine. One of the most celebrated incidents of adoption of black folk remedies by white medical authorities relates to smallpox. Smallpox inoculation (variolation) had been practiced in Africa by the early seventeenth century. Cotton Mather, the widely influential minister, writer, and scientist in early colonial history, is celebrated as a pioneer in promoting inoculation to prevent epidemic disease. It was one of his slaves, named Onesimus, who introduced Mather to this approach of inducing immunity to prevent smallpox. Yet Mather, not Onesimus, receives credit for having discovered and popularized this idea.

Often black health became a political issue in itself. Prevailing racial ideology emphasized poor health and disease among slaves as evidence of racial inferiority, and therefore justification for black enslavement. Conversely, when black Americans showed greater resistance to some diseases, whites saw it as validation for using them as manual laborers in harsh environments. Abolitionists used the deleterious effects of slavery on black health as evidence of the cruelty of slavery, and black abolitionists themselves often pursued healthcare fields as the best way to help African Americans.

Before the American Revolution, the belief that people of African descent comprised a separate race was widespread. Educated circles in the colonies proclaimed that blacks possessed a distinct physical biology and disease susceptibility. In his *Notes on Virginia* (1781–1782) Thomas Jefferson summarized this racial ethnology. A member of the South's slave-holding elite, Jefferson believed that nature had established "real distinctions" between the white and black races. These differences included physical attributes, such as hair, color, secretion, physical need for sleep, as well as differences in intellectual and reasoning capacity.

The belief in inherent racial differences surfaced with destructive effect during the yellow fever epidemic that ravaged cities beginning in the late 1700s. Yellow fever was a recurrent menace for the colonies and the early Republic United States. Until about 1800, the disease cropped up along the ports of the Northeast region. During the first half of the nineteenth century, yellow fever outbreaks occurred especially along the South Atlantic and Gulf Coast regions. The disease had been prevalent in the areas of West Africa from which North American slaves were taken. Also, yellow fever was endemic to the Caribbean region. For these reasons, black Americans exhibited a comparatively higher level of acquired immunity to yellow fever than did white populations. Medical historians and epidemiologists continue to question the widely held view throughout American history, supported by prominent medical historians, that the African and Caribbean populations and their descendants possessed an innate immunity to yellow fever. The opposing position stressed that black slaves acquired immunity from childhood exposure, and that this exposure occurred in subsequent generations of slave children throughout the historical course of slavery. This clash of scientific schools of thought was an undertone in the public hysteria surrounding the yellow fever epidemic that struck Philadelphia in 1793.

In the early 1790s, turmoil in the French West Indies resulted in a growing number of refugees from this area reaching the port of Philadelphia. As events that culminated in the Haitian Revolution gained momentum, Philadelphia became a pressure cooker of conflicting public sentiments surrounding the black presence in the nation's capital city. In the summer of 1793, cases of yellow fever began to appear throughout the city. By the end of August, authorities were encountering twenty cases a day of yellow fever sickness, and deaths from the disease began to mount into the hundreds.

In this age of premodern medicine, none of Philadelphia's medical or political leaders could pinpoint the cause of the disease. Some blamed rotting cargo piled on streets near the waterfront. Others blamed the refugees massing in the city. As the epidemic raged on, national political leaders, including President George Washington, avoided the city for several months. Some four thousand had died from yellow fever by the end of October. In early September, Philadelphia social reformer, physician, and politician Benjamin Rush (1745–1813), the most reputable physician during the Revolutionary Era, noticed that apparently no blacks had died from the disease. Rush began to encourage local blacks to assist with nursing the ill and removing the dead from the city.

In response to Rush's call, the prominent local black church leaders Richard Allen and Absalom Jones mobilized the efforts of the city's black community. The free black community's health providers were motivated by a strong sense of religious belief, as well as a willingness to assist the ill or injured, and honor and bury the dead. The healthcare networks of the slave communities throughout the South as well as in the northern free black communities were previously largely invisible to or undervalued by many slaveholders and their medical professionals. During the yellow fever epidemic, this black health network—along with its complex layers of agency and care for the ill—came to the surface.

In the end, blacks proved to be not as immune to yellow fever as whites had insisted. An estimated five hundred blacks died in the yellow fever outbreak. Moreover, even after their extraordinary public service, black Philadelphians were criticized in a widely circulated pamphlet by Mathew Carey,

A Short Account of the Malignant Fever. . . (1793). An Irish-born white and an influential publisher and philanthropist, Carey accused blacks of extorting and profiting from the victims of the scourge. In response, Allen and Jones published their own account of the virtuous work of their people called *A Narrative of the Proceedings of the Black People, During the Late Awful Calamity in Philadelphia in the Year 1793 and A Refutation of Some Censures Thrown Upon Them in Some Late Publications.*

Racial constructions of disease and susceptibility were widespread throughout the early Republic and antebellum nation. Medical writers and their articles in professional journals added pseudoscientific support to the white supremacist ideology of slaveholders and pro-slavery politicians. For example, in 1840 the U.S. federal census produced the first national statistics on the number of "insane" or "idiotic" by race and location. The census presented the number of "insane blacks" living in non-slaveholding states as strikingly high compared to those in slave states.

Pro-slavery science writers and business advocates leaped on these statistics, proclaiming they were clear scientific proof that freedom produced insanity in free black populations, while slavery prevented the disorder. More open-minded social researchers of the free North disputed this conclusion. Massachusetts physician and statistician Edward Jarvis published a methodic repudiation of this census report. Also, as years passed, black abolitionist-physician James McCune Smith and other abolitionists attacked insanity rates derived from the census report as filled with logical errors and, therefore, wholly invalid.

Thomas Jefferson and many of the Founding Fathers were part and parcel of the world of slave owners. As such, they turned a blind eye to the inhumanity of this economic system. However, as the nineteenth century wore on, black and white abolitionists, as well as outspoken fugitive slaves, were determined to expose the horrors of slavery. Renowned antislavery activists such as Harriet Tubman, Sojourner Truth, and Frederick Douglass made known the dreadful health conditions slaves in fields and plantation houses faced daily. These unhealthy places were just a stone's throw away from the stylish political buildings and large houses occupied by the new nation's Southern leaders.

By the mid-nineteenth century, the nation's boldest and most articulate abolitionist leaders and fugitive slaves began publishing tracts and narratives about the harsh reality of Southern slavery. Their aim was to educate the public about the wanton physical suffering and death the actions of slave owners caused slaves throughout the South's thousands of plantations. One such classic publication, *American Slavery As It Is: Testimony of a Thousand Witnesses* (1839) by abolitionist Theodore Dwight Weld, focused on the South's intentional destruction of slave health. Assembling thousands of Southern newspaper articles and extracting narratives, testimonies, and other factual pieces, Weld (1803–1895) and his wife, Angelina, and sister-in-law, Sarah, documented the gross mistreatment of slaves underway in the South. To counter critics who wanted to dismiss their survey as abolitionist propaganda, Weld employed a group of reputable abolitionists to verify their survey materials. Once published, *Slavery As It Is* quickly sold in the thousands. It presented detailed cases of brandings, shootings, overwork, whippings, and other "wanton cruelties" against slaves rife throughout the slave South. These hundreds of eyewitness accounts depicted the terrible plight of slaves as they barely clung to their lives, much less living healthfully.

From *Slavery As It Is* and other historical documents, it is clear that the medical care slaves received was frequently more harmful than helpful, while many slaves received no care or living resources beyond that suitable for bare subsistence. Slaves appearing to have terminal illnesses were often put in a bare isolated dwelling and left to die. One slave owner of some three hundred slaves in Huntsville, Alabama, in 1836 is reported to have said: "[A]fter employing a physician among them for some time, [I found] it was cheaper to lose a few negroes every year than to pay a physician." Another case an abolitionist highlighted involved the living quarters on the outskirts of a plantation for a sick slave woman owned by Francis Keen, a Virginia senator. The woman was barely clothed and living in a "hut [with] neither table, chair, nor chest—a stool and a rude fixture in one corner, were all its furniture. On this last [was] a little straw and a few old remnants of what had been bedding—all exceedingly filthy." At night another slave woman came to stay with her, as did slave children in the day, before she soon died.[3]

Slave owners, their family members, slave drivers, and even white men who owned no slaves meted out beatings and killings of slaves of all ages and both genders. Several incidents in northern Alabama recorded in *American Slavery As It Is* illustrated the violent social world that blacks faced in much of the South. One case described a white man named William Mosely and his assault on a slave near Courtland, Alabama. Mosely came home with a "bloody knife in his hand, having just stabbed a negro [sic] man. The negro was sitting quietly in a house in the village, keeping a woman company who had been left in charge of the house—when Mosely, passing along, went in and demanded his business there." When the black man did not answer to Mosely's satisfaction, "Mosely rushed upon him and stabbed him."[4]

In another incident in the same area of Alabama, a white man "shot a negro woman through the head; and put the pistol so close that her hair was singed." They had had some earlier "difficulty in his dealings" with her. Thompson buried the woman's body in a pile of logs, "she was discovered by the buzzards gathering around it." Also around the same time in northern Alabama, locals reported, two white men "found a fine looking negro man at 'Dandridge's Quarter,' without a pass; and flogged him so that he died in a short time. They were not punished." Then there are cases like these: "Col. Blocker's overseer attempted to flog a negro—he refused to be flogged; whereupon the overseer seized an axe, and cleft his skull. The Colonel justified it." And: "One Jones whipped a woman to death for 'grabbling' a potato hill. He owned 80 or 100 negroes."[5]

The growing public recognition of such inhumane treatment of bonded African Americans stoked an increasingly powerful antislavery sentiment throughout the North. Abolitionists and healthcare practitioners, black and white, focused increasingly on the fact that emancipation would be the only prescription to end such massive black suffering and preventable deaths. Still, in the decades immediately before the Civil War, the federal government constantly accommodated the political expansion of the slave system south and westward. Also, both federal and state government passed race-based laws restricting freed blacks from basic rights such as voting, serving on juries, or using public transportation. Northern states and territories passed laws that prohibited fugitive slaves from settling in these regions. Against this dismal political backdrop, a steady stream of black abolitionist physicians and healers merged into the antislavery movement. Many were informally trained doctors or folk healers, and virtually all were driven by strong religious and charitable beliefs. Some of the medical practitioners conducted their medical practice along with other professions such as publisher, educator, or business entrepreneur.

The more formally educated black abolitionist-physicians frequently wrote scientific tracts or public statements challenging popular white supremacist scientists of their day. These physicians aspired to prove the existence of a human biological spectrum on which people of all colors were equally endowed by nature as members within the human family. All of them combined abolition and healing in their work as the means to realize equality for the freed blacks and slaves throughout the nation.

Among the numerous outspoken black abolitionist-physicians were Martin Delaney and James McCune Smith. Martin Delaney (1812–1885) was a multifaceted thinker and entrepreneur drawn to medicine, but also to geography, journalism, oratory, and social activism. Admitted to Harvard Medical School, Delaney became a national political leader for free blacks. He became the country's chief advocate of emigration, a school of black activism that sought to link black Americans socially and commercially with the African homeland. Born in Charles Town, West Virginia, and spending much of his youth in central Pennsylvania, Delaney was one of the first blacks admitted to Harvard Medical School. Eventually he earned the role of a nationally prominent antislavery activist, working with Frederick Douglass to publish the *North Star*, Douglass's abolitionist newspaper.

In his medical activities, Delaney apprenticed with a number of white abolitionist doctors, including Andrew N. McDowell, Dr. F. Julius LeMoyne, and the Pittsburgh-based Dr. Joseph P. Gazzam. Delaney experienced both the national cholera epidemic of 1833 and the Pittsburgh epidemic of 1854. He focused on abolitionist newspaper work and public leadership of the northern free black communities. His book, *The Condition, Elevation, Emigration, and Destiny of the Colored People of the United States, Politically Considered* (1852), became a rallying cry for black emigration from the United States, and he moved to Canada in 1856. Three years later, he traveled to Liberia to explore the feasibility of black American emigration to that region. When the Civil War broke out, Delaney recruited blacks to fight for the U.S. Colored Troops (USCT). He became the first black field officer of the USCT to be commissioned major. In the final years of his life, Delaney practiced medicine in Charleston, South Carolina.

Similar to Martin Delaney, James McCune Smith (1813–1865) also became a physician and an antislavery leader simultaneously. Smith emerged from a network of black abolitionist intellectuals. Born in New York, he attended the African Free School, an historic seedbed for black educational leadership. Started by white abolitionists, this school educated the likes of black intellectuals and abolitionists Alexander Crummell, Henry Highland Garnet, and Samuel Ringgold Ward. Unable to obtain admission to numerous colleges in the United States, Smith earned college and medical degrees at the University of Glasgow and Scotland. He returned to New York after his education and started a pharmacy and a successful medical practice that served both white and black clients.

Smith became the physician for the Colored Orphans' Asylum, a charitable institution highly valued by the City's black community. In addition to his medical work, Smith was a devoted activist, educator, and scholar on behalf of the struggle for black equality. Among his numerous publications were his reflections on scientific matters involving race concepts, phrenology, and black American social elevation. Along with the likes of Martin Delaney and lay black abolitionist leaders such as Frederick Douglass, Smith was among the black intellectual vanguard. He and his colleagues produced writings, public discourse, and educational work that challenged the white racial ideology of his day.

Smith in particular attacked the antiblack assumptions of the new fields of natural heredity law and phrenology. He did this through public lectures, newspaper writings, and other published pieces. In 1837, Smith's essay, "The Fallacy of Phrenology," appeared in the nation's first black newspaper, *The Colored American*. Smith also published the first medical case report by a black physician: "Case of Ptyalism [i.e. excessive secretion of saliva] with Fatal Termination" (1840). As the years passed and the slavery issue heated up nationally, McCune Smith continued his antislavery activities. He went on to become professor of anthropology at Wilberforce University, in Ohio, but died only a few years afterward. Wilberforce, along with Lincoln University in Pennsylvania, were the nation's first black colleges.

Many other leading black abolitionist figures were also medical or nursing practitioners of some sort. Susie King Taylor (1848–1912) became perhaps the most prominent trained black nurse of the Civil War and late nineteenth century period. Born and raised in Georgia, Susie managed to gain an education and began working among freed blacks in Union-controlled areas of Georgia. Her relief work also took her to the South Carolina region at around the same time as Harriet Tubman was also actively serving in this area. Gradually Taylor's work in teaching and domestic tasks shifted to aiding military doctors nursing sick and wounded soldiers. In 1870, Taylor moved to Boston and became a full-time nurse for the Women's Relief Corps that assisted hospitals and soldiers. She wrote and self-published her memoirs, *My Life in Camp with the 33rd US Colored Troops* (1902).

Harriet Tubman (1822–1913) served in war relief in the Sea Island area of South Carolina, near Fort Wagner, where the U.S. Army maintained hospital facilities separately for white and black soldiers. Tubman worked to help

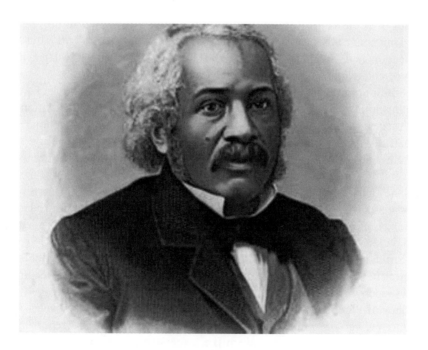

Figure 1.1. Dr. James McCune Smith (1813–1865). First African American physician with an M.D. degree.

Source: **Scanned image from Recollections of Seventy Years by Daniel Alexander Payne (1811–1893), published in 1888. Public domain.**

soldiers in this area, as did famed white nurse, Clara Barton, and Taylor. From about one year before and one year after the bloody Fort Wagner battle of July 1863, Tubman worked as a nurse and matron in a hospital in Beaufort, South Carolina. The facility served black soldiers and contraband blacks—that is, blacks who were slaves but who had managed to gain refuge with the Union forces. Tubman helped with direct care such as bathing the war-weary soldiers and dressing their wounds. She also assisted in sanitizing hospital facilities and burying the dead.

Harriet Tubman was steeped in the traditional folk medicine of the area and gained a reputation for her herbal remedies. Her concoctions seemed effective against diseases like dysentery and malaria. She was an illustrious agent and proselytizer for the Underground Railroad, abolitionist organizations, and humanitarian work among the Union troops and freed populations during Civil War. By the end of the 1880s, Tubman was known as the "Moses" of her people. She spent her final years in her hometown of Auburn, New York. There she lived with very little personal funds, working to her last days trying to establish a home for the elderly and disabled.

Like Harriet Tubman, Sojourner Truth became a health caretaker for the Union soldiers and newly freed black populations during the Civil War era. In the early years of the war, Truth assisted the black recruits who were forming the famous 54th Regiment of the U.S. Colored Troops. At the war's close she worked with the National Freedmen's Relief Association in Washington, DC. In September of 1865, a few months after the war ended, she took on duties at the Freedmen's Hospital. There she assisted with the health of the soldiers and black free populations suffering from extreme destitution. While performing duties at Freedmen's, Truth also began a battle against segregated public streetcars.

In a broader historical context, Harriet Tubman and Sojourner Truth's holistic care approach foreshadowed the strong hold Christian spiritualism maintained in black America, even in the twentieth century and beyond. Both women were avowed Christian spiritualists. The holistic spiritualist approach of these women meant that they believed the physical fate of the suffering person under their care was linked to that person's willingness to believe their health was destined by God. Spiritualism began as a movement in the nineteenth century that swept through many Southern cities, especially New Orleans. The persistence of the spiritualist worldview in black health history and in current-day black health rests with its power to address the individual's deepest sense of psychological and physical need. Spiritualism motivates the sick and the healers to connect their healing to a more just order of the world in which they live. In other words, healing the sick is necessary to improve society as a whole. Caregivers and sufferers or patients can experience spiritualism without the necessity of either a formal place of worship or a formal place of healthcare. Thus, the spiritualism personified in the care work of Tubman and Truth expanded throughout subsequent generations in black communities.

Overall, by the mid-nineteenth century, the health of black Americans carried the deep scars of institutional slavery. Nonetheless, black populations grew as they outmaneuvered the heavy odds against survival that the slavery system had meted out to them. Most black healthcare practitioners through the second half of the nineteenth century were abolitionists, medical entrepreneurs, folk healers, and spiritual caregivers. Many were motivated by Christian aspirations, folk medicine, and humanitarian ideals. Fueled by so many streams of motivation, their healthcare and charitable work flowed into the black American's broader quest for social equality. Indeed, the medical men and women of black America through the Civil War period were in keeping with what historian Cedric Robinson has called the Afro-Christian core culture of black Americans. This core culture in later decades would inspire the modern black health equality movement as well as the civil rights struggle for full citizenship and equality.

Chapter Two

Battling for Life in the Civil War and Nadir Eras

The Civil War and Reconstruction brought about a revolutionary change in the political status of black Americans. These events ushered in emancipation, citizenship, male suffrage, and other constitutional protections for black Americans—at least in the written laws of the land. However, on the day-to-day level, blacks still had to endure living as a subordinate race. Throughout the nation, many in the general public disdained these nearly four million newly freed slaves in their midst. Furthermore, the wartime destruction and refugee populations the Civil War left behind had produced social upheaval and epidemics that killed both whites and blacks. While most white political and social leaders expected their own race to survive, many whites believed the opposite fate awaited blacks.

Before the Civil War, cities relied on dispensaries and charity hospitals to care for the sick and disabled. Great masses of people living in large cities were housed in unventilated, congested tenement rooms. In these dense population centers, many with black neighborhoods, both sewage and water supplies were unsanitary. Diseases such as dysentery, cholera, and tuberculosis were widespread. The influx of poor European immigrants during the 1840s and 1850s intensified in these same cities, especially in the northeast and mid-Atlantic states. From 1845 to 1855 alone, some three million immigrants flowed into the nation's northern states and western territories primarily from countries like Germany, Ireland, Italy, and Wales. This immigrant population crowded into the same unhealthy urban areas as did the free blacks.

During the antebellum period, there was little scientific understanding of diseases like tuberculosis and yellow fever to guide hospital doctors. Therefore, healthcare facilities in cities functioned mostly as poorhouses, asylums, and custodial buildings. Throughout mid-nineteenth-century industrial America, the local wealthy and other charitable segments supported these facilities. Although the care they provided was inefficient and overtaxed, these hospitals and dispensaries nonetheless eased the suffering of the urban poor. They also strengthened community cohesion of their particular ethnic and religious benefactors and patients.

Once the Civil War broke out and the conflict expanded, city hospitals, dispensaries, and physicians throughout the North and in war zones faced urgent emergency-care challenges. In the North, transporting and massing together hundreds of thousands of new soldiers and civilian military workers created conditions ripe for public health menaces. Once troop movements and battles began in full, a horrendous scale of death, destruction, and casualties were unleashed. Tens of thousands of freed slaves, wounded soldiers, and refugees flooded into already crowded cities and towns, especially those located in Union war zones. Some of these slaves were involved in the Underground Railroad, the secret network to assist runaway slaves plotting individual escape. But now they had the expanding cover of battle conditions to facilitate their escape from plantation and slave patrols. Initially the military camps, as well as the hospitals and dispensaries in Northern and military regions, were unprepared for such a flood of black slaves, black soldiers, and other refugees. The escaping and abandoned slaves settled near or inside Union camps and battle lines. Known as "contrabands," these freed slaves were considered confiscated property by Union military authorities. The Union forces would tolerate these new arrivals, but initially had no plans to help them physically survive.

The contrabands organized themselves into "contraband camps," or settlements. Inside these communities, networks of self-reliance became key. Food and group shelter, folk health practices, and religious activism and leadership were garnered in the same method that had helped blacks survive plantation slavery for decades before the Union troops and camps had arrived. As the Civil War dragged on and military zones expanded, the federal government faced growing pressure of wounded and disease-sickened soldiers, escaping and abandoned local slaves, and other civilian refugees. In effect, the government had to take up the health equality ideal.

This new public health mission reflected the urgent intention of federal and Union Army leaders to subdue the Confederate and upper South border states. The federal government and Union Army resolved to provide healthcare and sanitary resources for each segment of the War-affected population, including black Americans, 95 percent of whom were slaves. Caught in the national civil strife, free and slave black Americans did not just rely on government and military healthcare aid to survive the physical and biological turmoil the Civil War had unleashed. They also depended on their traditional community self-reliance, as well as charitable relief programs provided by white and free black relief organizations. At the War's height, and in its immediate aftermath, benevolent organizations led by the American Missionary Association worked directly with contraband camps and other black refugee sites.

During the War, government and military relief workers in Washington, DC, encountered a stream of black refugees arriving in different parts of the city. Washington became a "haven of refuge" for emancipated slaves, fleeing the revenge of Confederates and harsh living conditions in war-damaged areas. Slavery, a mainstay throughout the District of Columbia, was not abolished in this city until 1862. Therefore, initially newly freed blacks and other civilian war victims converged with local slave populations of the city. Consequently there was a strong backlash from the city's whites toward the thousands of freed blacks entering the city. One local white political leader sent a memorial to Congress imploring it to "provide safeguard against converting this city into an asylum for free Negroes, a population undesirable in any community."[1]

An estimated six million soldiers were either sickened or wounded as a result of the military combat of the Civil War. The death toll overall from the conflict is estimated to have been from 650,000 to 850,000. In the years immediately after the War, Dr. Robert Reyburn, a white Union surgeon born in Ireland, led the Freedmen's Bureau's relief commission for the city of Washington. Reyburn estimated that of the approximately 31,500 blacks residing in Washington and Georgetown in 1866, about two-thirds had an ailment of some sort. The black and white destitute crowding the District of Columbia needed the Bureau's aid desperately.

With the support of local benevolent organizations, and through Reyburn's commission, the Freedmen's Bureau provided the public relief supplies. This aid consisted of groceries, clothing, fuel, medicines, and small sums of cash. According to Reyburn, to incoming freed blacks, the city seemed a place of heavenly relief. Temporary quarters and camps were organized in different parts of the city for the black newcomers. One site, Camp Barker, was essentially a contraband settlement and a soldier relief area consisting of a few frame buildings. In 1862, a combination of patriotism and interracial altruism led to the camp's transformation into the Freedmen's Hospital and Asylum. Doctors Reyburn, the hospital's surgeon general from 1868 to 1875, and Charles B. Purvis, one of Freedmen's first African American surgeons in chief, were key figures in the growth of the hospital. Placed under the control of the Freedmen's Bureau in 1865, in its early years Freedmen's Hospital served an interracial patient base, including several hundred mental and severely disabled patients. To provide a place to continue care of these people, the head of the Freedmen's Bureau, General O. O. Howard, ordered the construction of new buildings on the grounds of Howard University, and Freedmen's eventually became the teaching hospital for the university's medical school.

Like Reyburn, Charles B. Purvis, M.D., described the origins of Freedmen's Hospital as a breakthrough for charity. The son of the famous black abolitionist and entrepreneur Robert Purvis, Charles Purvis devoted his medical career to the Hospital. He served as one of the handful of official doctors designated "colored person's surgeons" at the Freedmen's Bureau from 1865 to 1867, and in 1881 was appointed by President Chester A. Arthur as the surgeon in charge of Freedmen's Hospital. Purvis noted from the moment the freed people appeared in the District, "[d]isease early made its appearance." The freed blacks coming into the District were like a needy person "guided by some altruistic power . . . embrac[ing] every opportunity to escape from his bondage to the seat of government." This black American "was not encouraged in his endeavor, really not desired; still, in numbers he came. He was poor and homeless. Men, women and children of all conditions infested the city." According to Purvis, the "presence of this helpless mass soon became a subject of serious consideration," which had led to the establishment of Freedmen's Hospital.[2]

In its early years, Freedmen's was under the leadership of Lieutenant Colonel Alexander T. Augusta (1825–1890). A surgeon and veteran of the Civil War, Dr. Augusta was the nation's first black medical professor. During the Reconstruction years and after, he became an important mentor to black medical trainees at the Hospital, and to black medical professionals generally. Dr. Augusta was one of America's early black medical achievers—that is, someone who gained a national reputation among black Americans for representing the highest ideals of a profession and earned national esteem. Likewise, Freedmen's Hospital became a touchstone of medical scientific achievement for black Americans.

By 1879, Freedmen's dispensaries provided annual treatment to about 2,270 outpatients and issued some 4,000 prescriptions. When the Freedmen's Bureau closed in 1872, many anticipated that Freedmen's Hospital would close, as well. However, due to skillful agitation by the likes of Dr. Reyburn, the Hospital's first surgeon in chief, Congress had authorized a special bill and administrative committee to keep the hospital operating. Over the next few decades, Freedmen's rose to prominence as the nation's first institution dedicated to the medical treatment of black Americans.

Serving as surgeon in charge of Freedmen's from 1881 to 1894, Purvis believed that Freedmen's was the most humanitarian answer to the formerly enslaved race's longing for tolerance and charity. In his role as a leader in medical education and hospital care for the nation's blacks, Purvis encouraged the graduates of Freedmen's Hospital to realize that medicine was advancing rapidly. He also disdained health and moral practices exhibited by many blacks, especially youth, as precarious. He viewed improving the health of black Americans as the special responsibility of the black physician, but he also tied better health practices to higher morality and racial improvement. For example, with regard to drinking and smoking, Purvis admonished "[t]here can be no perpetuity for our institutions; there can be no future of the race if these practices, I may say crimes, go unchallenged and unchecked."[3]

Thus, to its early medical administrators, the first years of Freedmen's Hospital reflected the fruition of the Civil War ideals of freedom and equality for black Americans. This idea, that charitable hospital and medical care for the black poor originated during the tumultuous decades between the Civil War and the end of the nineteenth century, became the public memory most often proselytized by the leaders of these institutions. Soon, other black hospitals developed throughout other parts of the nation. But Freedmen's was the beacon for them. As eminent black medical scholar William Montague Cobb wrote in celebration of Freedmen's one hundredth anniversary in 1962: "Both the philosophy of [Freedmen's] origin and continued existence . . . has never been divorced from the concept of freedom."[4]

In the decades immediately following Reconstruction, public consternation about black health continued nationwide. The acceleration of this public crisis was due to several converging forces. First, the Compromise of 1876 meant that federal military protection for blacks was withdrawn from throughout the Reconstruction South. This opened the door for a wave of racial violence, including lynching propagated against blacks to disrupt their community stability and political participation. Second, a new form of social racism took hold. Social Darwinist medical and scientific arguments and ideologies rationalized the poverty and neglectful living and health conditions blacks experienced. Anthropological scholars and medical leaders spread ideas purporting the inherent inferiority of the black race. Doctors and academic leaders, mostly throughout the white South, predicted the inevitable demise of the black race. These racial ideas discouraged reform efforts to improve public health and economic conditions that freed slaves and other postwar black populations endured.

Third, the U.S. Supreme Court issued its infamous *Plessy v. Ferguson* decision in 1896, which established the "separate but equal" doctrine that held segregation was constitutional if blacks had equal facilities provided to them. In practice, black facilities were far from equal, but this principle became the legal foundation for the spread of Jim Crow segregation laws throughout the entire South and many communities in the North as well. The combination of Jim Crow laws, politics, anti-black violence, and race science resulted in historians characterizing the post-Reconstruction decades as the Nadir for black American political history. In many respects, black health plumbed the depths, as well.

From the onset of the post-Reconstruction Era, Southern public health offices, hospitals, federal census surveys, and physicians who treated black patients reported substantial black and white health disparities. In 1881, the Memphis Board of Health reported that while the city's black and white populations were virtually equal in size, in that year there were 806 black deaths, compared to 665 deaths for whites. As for children under the age of five, some 356 black children had died that same year compared to 204 white children. Birth rates for blacks were down, as well.

The higher rates of sickness for blacks struck fear throughout many of the nation's white city politicians and civic leaders. At its annual public health conference in 1887, the Kentucky Board of Health addressed the critical plight of the South's black residents. One of the city's leading white religious figures told the conference that the health situation facing blacks living in Southern cities was urgent. The "colored people are resorting to the towns and cities, and falling victims to all the diseases that fester in the lowest elements of those cities." Citing municipal health statistics, city leaders in the South were pessimistic about the future for blacks: "The ravages of disease are increasing with a fearful ratio among the colored people, and as yet no signs appear of relief arising up from among themselves. . . . We see the problem of the negro's [*sic*] future dark with gloom."[5]

Such pessimism about black health was not just segregationist rhetoric. In New Orleans between 1860 and 1880, the annual death rates for blacks ranged between 32 and 81 per thousand compared to 5 and 39 per thousand for whites. Of the 1,000 black infants born in this city in the year 1880, an estimated 450 died. Outbreaks of diseases in the black city sections such as cholera and smallpox were constant. Historians attribute these high death rates to overcrowded, unventilated tenements and shacks located within unsanitary conditions, as well as inadequate food and drinking water in the household of poor blacks and whites.

When the New Orleans Board of Health issued its 1880 report, it called black health one of the city's most serious problems. Its explanation for the high black mortality rates was a mixture of Southern racism, ignorance about health attitudes, and scattershot observations. It stated that the excessive black mortality rates were caused by: "(a) improvidence in living, irregular habits; poor diets; (b) neglect of the sick; indifference to medical aid; neglect of vaccination; (c) crowding and imperfect ventilation; (d) less vital power or capacity to resist the ravages of diseases; [and] (e) ignorance of, and violation of, physiological and sanitary laws."[6]

With mortality and sickness rates for blacks during the 1880s and 1890s appallingly high, the question of whether the black race could survive into the twentieth century actually became a national public issue. At the same time national developments in race relations were troubling to American public leaders. Federal courts were under pressure to weigh in on the citizenship issues blacks were facing; the federal military was expanding into foreign, non-white lands; and blacks were restless in the South and beginning to look to other parts of the nation to settle. Responding to these cross-pressures involving national racial and political identity, leading anthropologists, economists, and physicians interpreted the relatively dismal public health data concerning blacks as the empirical proof for their ideas that blacks possessed distinct anatomical traits and disease susceptibilities.

Interpreting their findings through a social Darwinist lens, many of the nation's medical science and political economy authorities proclaimed that physical traits set the Negro "race" apart from European and Asian races of peoples. As part of their distorted pseudoscientific worldview, these public officials, popular scientists, and medical writers also asserted that slavery had been a protective institution for black slaves. In their view, emancipation and the Civil War constitutional amendments granting blacks political citizenship had thrown off the benefits that the slave system had provided America's blacks. According to these scientists and commentators, blacks by themselves lacked the moral capacity to supply their own safe housing and other economic needs.

The economic statistician Frederick Hoffman wrote one of the most influential studies trumpeting black racial decline. Published by the American Economic Association, Hoffman's *The Race Traits and Tendencies of the American Negro* (1896) amplified the Old South physician's beliefs in black racial inferiority. According to Hoffman, "the colored population is gradually parting with the virtues . . . developed under the regime of slavery." He cautioned that blacks possessed "an immense amount of immorality" and therefore, the spread of syphilis and tuberculosis throughout their numbers was inevitable.[7]

Public health departments around the nation working with black populations seemed to reinforce the medical and social science writers who spelled doom for black Americans. Most public health agencies around the nation emphasized that tuberculosis was the most persistent and deadly health problem facing blacks. Annual vital statistics and public health reports reflected marked racial disparities in TB rates. For example, according to U.S. Census reports on death rates in 1900, the overall TB mortality rate for whites in registered areas was 174 per 100,000 population. By comparison, the TB death rate for blacks in Baltimore was 448; in New York, 503; in Washington, DC, 514; and in Boston, 742. Many doctors and public health workers, black and white alike, and mostly in the North and Midwest, were aware that certain environmental conditions seemed to increase TB case rates. These included congested housing, impoverished neighborhoods, crowded workplaces, and ignorance about lay practices that increased the risk of spreading the disease, such as spitting. Many health authorities in liberal, largely northern municipal settings proclaimed an interest in reducing these conditions in their respective cities and towns. However, concrete measures could only proceed if they could locate and work with black healthcare workers to implement them.

In the South, most white public health authorities and physicians were concerned with high black TB rates from a position of self-interest. They feared that the disease could easily pass from black carriers to white households and communities. In Southern cities and towns, blacks possibly infected with TB had regular contacts with whites—as domestics and cooks, for example. In 1910, the *Journal of the American Medical Association* published an article by the Richmond physician Thomas W. Murrell on "The Negro as a Health Problem." Expressing ideas widely held among his Southern white colleagues, Murrell remarked that blacks without slavery were an alarming menace to both himself and society at large. According to Murrell, a black person, "as a rule [is] but a sorry specimen . . . [m]orality among these people is almost a joke . . . and venereal disease [is] well-nigh universal." Without slavery, blacks were now "free indeed," Murrell wrote, "free to get drunk with cheap political whiskey and to shiver in the cold . . . free never to bathe, and to sleep in hovels where God's sunlight and air could not penetrate." Furthermore, a black man was "absolutely free to gratify his every sexual impulse; to be infected with every loathsome disease and to infect his ready and willing companions—and he did it—he did it all. The result is the negro [*sic*] of 1909, the negro of today."[8]

In the opening decade of the twentieth century, state and local public health agencies, hospitals, and physician reports portrayed blacks as a hazardous population both to themselves and to the white public at large. However, like the antebellum census surveys, these reports were haphazardly collected, misinterpreted, or simply ignored if they pointed toward equal susceptibility or infection rates regardless of race. For example, although high rates of venereal disease reported for blacks were a critical issue for white medical and public health leaders around the country, military health surveys of some 60,000 black and white troops in 1904—some of whom had served in the Philippines, Puerto Rico, and Cuba—indicated that the rate of VD in whites had been about one-quarter higher than black rates.

Other health authorities observed that historic exposures to certain diseases led to lower rates among the black population, as in the case of malaria and yellow fever. However, as black leaders at the Atlanta University Negro Conference in 1906 discussed, the public and many of the nation's health leaders largely ignored such statistics and disease patterns. Instead, up until the start of World War I, most national public health, medical authorities, and politicians involved in contentious race relations in their districts relied on observations and surveys of Southern white physicians and health departments. Moreover, many Southern health and public authorities believed that blacks lacked the moral control and community order necessary to avoid high disease rates.

By the start of the twentieth century, the black American contributions to the War for the Union and Reconstruction reforms had all but receded from the national memory. At the same time, fatalism about the decline of the black race was widespread. While many whites still believed that blacks were incapable of helping themselves, black Americans slowly but effectively built their own, largely self-reliant health and social welfare resources. Anti-black discrimination endemic to Jim Crow institutional life restricted these group efforts, especially throughout the South. Nonetheless, to the youthful, increasingly educated black American national community, physicians, hospitals, and medical training institutions were vital to their race's collective survival. Indeed, black and racially liberal America expected that a new black professional class would take on the leadership of the nation's African Americans. Consequently, together they started black medical schools, hospitals, and community health reform programs. These seminal initiatives, in turn, helped to produce a rising, educated and modern black healthcare sector.

In the Nadir period, the prohibition against black entrants to the nation's white medical schools and professional associations was virtually ironclad. Doctors in America were struggling for professional esteem. Compared to the clinically focused doctors and medical education in France, U.S. physicians were organized around a chaotic stew of for-profit practices and medical school training, approaches lacking a core clinical approach. The health reforms and sanitary knowledge that flourished as a result of the Civil War and Reconstruction experiences had helped to push the medical profession more toward pragmatic and effective approaches to disease engagement.

Nonetheless, during the Nadir of race relations, whites were dismissive of blacks or women participating as teachers or students in the nation's leading medical schools and hospitals. Many white male medical professionals believed that such participation would threaten their efforts to earn broader status as a cultural elite. They viewed women, black Americans, and other ethnic minorities seeking to enter the medical profession as potentially tarnishing the scientific and professional prestige of white physicians. Moreover, according to popular white racial etiquette, admitting blacks into white medical schools and hospitals to work among white patients was out of the question. In 1906, Charles H. Frazier, M.D., dean of the University of Pennsylvania's medical school, made this point succinctly in rejecting an application from a black youth, William J. Harvey Jr. of Atlanta:

> I am afraid that your being colored would handicap you very seriously in this institution, inasmuch as in all our clinical work the students are brought in

close contact with the patients, and very many patients object to being examined by, or being exhibited before colored students. [9]

By contrast, certain government public health agencies, Freedmen's Hospital, and other black hospitals and medical schools were consciously striving
to cultivate more black medical practitioners. These institutions and black
medical professionals formed a common stream of hospital-based medical
activity and community service for the nation's black communities. One
black physician in particular enabled these new black clinically trained doctors and nurses to work at the innovative edge of American medicine: surgeon Daniel Hale Williams.

At the turn of the twentieth century, specialists in the field of surgery, in
particular, became some of the earliest medical providers dedicated to clinical training of their practitioners and standardized arrangements for surgical
operations. The young talented surgeons learned that for science-based medicine and hospitals to be successful, the clinical practitioner had to adhere to
each and all aspects of professional hospital care and medical treatment. In
accord with this ideal, in 1891 Williams founded the Provident Hospital and
Training School for Nurses in Chicago, so that black and white doctors alike
could practice clinical medicine in a modernized hospital setting. Organized
as a multiracial enterprise, this was the nation's first black-controlled hospital. Williams, like his modern physician peers nationwide, knew that the
professionalization of nursing was vital to advance hospital-based medicine.
Therefore, Williams also organized Provident to serve as a training center for
nurses. Initially the institution had a significant number of white patients. But
as the hospital's surrounding community became increasingly concentrated
with black residents, the majority (over 90 percent) of the hospital's patients
soon became black.

Like Freedmen's Hospital in Washington, Provident became black Chicago's pivotal center for the training of physicians and nurses, on one hand, and
medical care for the city's blacks, on the other. By the start of World War I,
all of Provident's nurses were black, as were most of its staff physicians.
Between them the Freedmen's Bureau, Freedmen's Hospital, and Provident
Hospital trained and distributed into the nation's black communities a steady
stream of expertly prepared black medical and nursing achievers.

At the same time as Dr. Williams and his hospital improvement campaigns were gaining momentum, female black medical figures were also
emerging from Freedmen's Bureau activities forging links with progressive
hospitals, including Provident. Rebecca Lee Crumpler (1831–1895) was one
such physician. Born in Delaware, she was raised by an aunt who was a
popular caretaker of the local sick. From this experience, Lee decided to start
doing nursing tasks for doctors. Eventually she graduated from the New
England Female Medical College in 1860, becoming the first formally edu-

cated African American woman physician. Eventually she broadened her practice to center on family and community service. Following the Civil War, Lee located to Richmond, Virginia, and worked for the Freedmen's Bureau among the destitute, which included an estimated thirty thousand black people. Crumpler dedicated her book, *A Book of Medical Discourses* (1883), to mothers and nurses. The first medical text published by a black American woman, it focused on the health and medical problems of children and women.

Another black woman physician of significance was a younger peer of Crumpler, Rebecca J. Cole (1846–1922). Born in Philadelphia, Cole attended the Woman's Medical College of Pennsylvania (now Drexel University's medical school). In her fifty years of medical practice, she led relief work and ran homes for the needy. Early in her career, Cole worked at the New York Infirmary for Women and Children under the famous Dr. Elizabeth Blackwell. The hospital employed Cole for the position of sanitary inspector, to visit poor patients in their homes and to give poor mothers special instruction on infant care and maintaining healthy homes. Dr. Blackwell described Cole as an "intelligent young coloured physician [who] carried on this work with tact and care. Experience of its results serve to show that the establishment of such a department would be a valuable addition to every hospital."[10]

Both Crumpler's and Cole's careers demonstrated formally trained black medical practitioners were just as comfortable as white practitioners in incorporating the scientific aspects of their profession into their careers. However, even as medicine became more clinically specialized and the upper-class social prestige of doctors grew throughout the nation, black medical professionals like Cole and Crumpler directed their skills toward broader community health needs, working among the newly emancipated black masses and black community overall. In the following decades and centuries, there was a continuous stream of technically competent black medical and nursing professionals who added to the nation's medical science heritage. But at the same time, these new black medical professionals were steadfastly devoted to the health equality ideal.

Among black medical practitioners of the late nineteenth century, Daniel Hale Williams became renowned for exemplifying the ideals of medical science and racial egalitarianism. In 1893, Williams conducted an operation at Provident that created a public stir in Chicago. A young black man by the name of James Cornish had been stabbed in a fight at a bar. His chest wound bled profusely, and Williams had to surgically open Cornish's chest and expose the heart. Prior to this incident, operating on the heart had been considered highly dangerous. Williams deftly sutured the membrane over the heart called the pericardium. Opening of the chest cavity had usually caused patients to succumb to infections. However, because he used modern antiseptic techniques, Williams's operation beat those odds.

Following his operation, Cornish remained in the hospital for fifty-one days; and went on to fully recover. The local press gave Williams's feat coverage; however, the medical publications carried articles of later cases claiming to have completed the first such operation, in effect obscuring Williams's groundbreaking achievement. Williams himself managed to correct the record a few years later in his 1897 article, "Stab Wound of the Heart and Pericardium—Suture of the Pericardium—Recovery—Patient Alive Three Years Afterward," which appeared in the *Medical Record.*

Most formally trained medical doctors in these last decades of the nineteenth century still lacked standardized clinical and diagnostic training. During this time doctors and hospitals were struggling to win public support and legal authority. Therefore, Williams brought to his peer black healthcare practitioners and supporters a wide-ranging perspective of the invaluable importance of medicine based on scientific principles and efficient patient care. He believed that effective medical treatment and recovery in the hospital required the highest standards of diagnosis, clinical procedures, and bedside care. He also stressed the importance of sterilization of hospital rooms and equipment, as well as sanitary environments for patients in their recovery settings.

Williams was well in step with modern medicine trends; in fact, he exemplified them as he headed initiatives to implement modern surgery, medical education, and nurses' training at both his Provident Hospital in Chicago and later Freedmen's Hospital. In 1894, he assumed the position as chief surgeon at Freedmen's Hospital. Under Williams's influence, the hospital finally emerged from being considered essentially the "poor man's retreat" into a genuine hospital. That year under Dr. Williams's leadership, Provident opened its training school for nurses. The hospital also started an ambulance unit of horse-drawn wagons that moved about the city streets and neighborhoods. Finally, at Freedmen's, Williams led the organization of the hospital into specific departments to match specific patient problems and treatment needs—that is, surgical, medical, genitourinary, gynecological, obstetrical, throat and chest, and dermatology departments. Williams's professional reputation expanded as he served as an organizer of black physicians, as well as a teacher in the nation's black medical schools. In 1913, Williams also became a charter member of, and the only black physician in, the American College of Surgeons.

The nation's broader black healthcare sector increasingly benefited from the black medical leaders who had backgrounds tied to Freedmen's Bureau health work, or Freedmen's and Provident Hospitals. In 1895, Williams and eleven other black medical professionals met at the Atlanta and Cotton States International Exhibition and formed a professional organization, the National Negro Medical Association of Physicians, Surgeons, Dentists, and Pharmacists—later known as the National Medical Association (NMA). Williams served as its copresident with physician and dentist Robert F. Boyd. The group designed the association as a body that would uplift black practitioners of medicine—and then, as an organization, work to uplift their entire race. The NMA provided the organizational base for black physicians, since they were excluded from membership in the American Medical Association. These black professionals demanded that society strive for health equality across the races, whether or not the South was ready to deal with the question of political equality for blacks. In the Post-Reconstruction Era, blacks in both the South and the urban North intrinsically knew they had to win the battle for health regardless of their political fate, over which they had only limited, if any, control.

Under the spreading influence of these health activists and organizations, in the 1880s and 1890s, dozens of other black hospitals as well as medical and nursing training programs sprouted in black communities in both the South and the North. These facilities trained and employed black physicians, dentists, pharmacists, and nurses. As of 1906, there were five medical schools specifically founded for training black physicians, pharmacists, and nurses.

Outside of Washington, DC, Meharry Medical College of Walden University in Nashville was the most important black medical training institution. Established by the Methodist Episcopal Church, this school became one of the two black medical schools that trained the largest numbers of black doctors and health professionals. In 1906, it had a faculty of 34 members as well as 320 medical students, 88 dental students, 35 pharmaceutical students, and 6 nursing students. Since its inception in 1876, the school had graduated a total of 733 doctors, 74 dentists, 85 pharmacists, and 15 nurses. The second medical school educating the largest number of blacks was the Howard University Medical School. Funded by the government, it was founded in 1867 and centered at the Freedmen's Hospital. As of 1906, Howard had 147 medical students, 31 dental students, and 26 pharmaceutical students, and it had graduated 543 physicians, 67 dentists, and 108 pharmacists.

Third among this group of leading early black medical schools was Leonard Medical School of Shaw University in Raleigh, North Carolina. Founded under the control of the Northern Baptists, in 1882, its enrollment in 1906 encompassed 147 medical students and 31 pharmaceutical students. Since its inception, the school had graduated 236 in medicine and 64 in pharmacy. In New Orleans, Flint Medical College opened in 1889 under the auspices of the Methodist Episcopal Church as part of New Orleans University. With a faculty of eleven, by 1906 this institution had graduated a total of 73 students in medicine, 8 in pharmacy, and 26 in nursing. In Kentucky, the Louisville National Medical College began operating in 1887. Its enrollment in 1906 included 47 medical students and 3 nursing students. Its overall graduates numbered 83 medical graduates, 1 pharmaceutical graduate, and

11 nurse graduates. In addition to these five schools, Knoxville College had started a medical college in 1895, but it closed after a short period of operation, and graduated only 2 medical students.

This small cluster of black medical schools was responsible for significant growth of blacks within the medical professions. In 1890, the U.S. Census Bureau reported there were 909 black physicians, 115 of them women. By 1900, this total number had increased over 90 percent. There were 1,734 black physicians, 160 of whom were female. Likewise, the census listed 120 black dentists in 1890. By 1900, this number had increased 77 percent to 212. Pharmacists were also a key component of the black medical sector. In 1890, there were 139 listed in the census as pharmacists or retail "dealers in drugs and medicine." By 1900, this number approximated three hundred.[11]

As urban America entered its Progressive Age, black reform leaders nationwide, believing in the social leadership of black doctors, nurses, and hospital organizers, endorsed medical idealism, the belief that progress in medical science and professions resulted in broad social advances for all of society. Beginning in 1896, the leaders of Atlanta University, which eventually included W. E. B. Du Bois, organized the annual Atlanta University Conference for the Study of Negro Problems. The goals at the heart of these national gatherings were social progressivism and black self-reliance. "The Conference above all reiterates its well known attitude toward this and all other social problems," the 1906 report stated. "[T]he way to make conditions better is . . . the systematic study of the Negro problems. . . . [Thus we] ask all aid and sympathy for the work of this conference in such study."[12]

The 1906 conference focused on the theme "The Health and Physique of the Negro American." Leading scholars, educators, civic activists, and social leaders from many parts of the nation attended, and the published conference proceedings included surveys and letters from health facilities and agencies located throughout the nation. The Conference attendees stressed that while blacks were still in dire need of better hospitals and medical care, the black medical professional sector and its hospitals were progressing. Their data revealed that the number of black doctors and medical establishments were significantly larger than reflected in official statistics. It reported 40 black hospitals, 1,500 black physicians, and some 200 black drugstores. Also they proudly reported that black-owned drugstores amounted to investments valued at a half million dollars, and they employed 800 workers.

Although highly idealistic upon graduating from medical school, each new black professional, regardless of his or her field, looked toward an unpredictable future. Race obstacles could appear at any level and at any stage in their careers. The Atlanta conference on black health reported about the recent experience of a bright black dentist. At first, he was selected to head international dental clinics for an important dental profession body.

However, once the group discovered he was black, he had to resign. The 300 black pharmacists in the nation at this time were confined to employment mostly in "colored drugstores."

While the educated and economic elite sectors of black America struggled to gain a foothold inside the nation's medical institutions, self-care through popular means remained the dominant "medical care" for typical black folk. For the masses of black Americans, healthcare resources were most usually rendered by informal means. During the late nineteenth and early twentieth centuries, drawing from the centuries-old culture of the slavery era, black folk or "roots" healing remained widespread throughout Southern black communities. These men and women healers used herbs, roots, and other natural substances to stem both physical and mental ills the individual had experienced. Zora Neale Hurston described root doctors and conjurers as similar: "'Roots' is the southern Negro's term for folk-doctoring by herbs and prescriptions," she once explained, "and by extension, and because all Hoodoo doctors cure by roots, it may be used as a synonym for Hoodoo."[13]

Flowing from the same traditional folk cultural roots, black midwives were still common throughout Southern black communities, as they were in white Southern, rural, and immigrant communities across the nation. Several forces held together the continuing widespread prevalence of lay midwife practices. Women within traditional cultures were comfortable fulfilling their historical roles as midwives, and likewise, birthing mothers were comfortable with their care. Moreover, delivery by physicians trained in obstetrics was still in its technical infancy. For most working-class women, hospital or physician deliveries were neither practically nor cheaply available.

Finally, even as hospital and physician deliveries gained wider acceptance among educated and urban female populations, women in black communities throughout the South were facing the thickening wall of Jim Crow discrimination. This wall combined with traditional patriarchal restrictions prevented them from either participating fully or escaping subordinate roles in all public institutions—from voting booths, to public schools and universities, to hospitals. Thus, access to hospital deliveries or physician care for most black women in the years before World War I was not the norm in the South's most heavily black-populated regions.

Along with black physicians and folk practitioners and midwives, black professional nurses made up the final vital one-third of the core black healthcare network. Strong social currents, stemming back to the pre–Civil War years, flowed together to orient aspirations of blacks, mostly women, toward the nursing profession. First, during the centuries of slavery and quasifree life in the North, a strong tradition had grown among black women as leaders in family, community, and social organizations. Second, public memory of the relief work and nursing activities of women like Harriet Tubman, Sojourner Truth, and Susie King had been exemplary to younger generations. The dedication of illustrious women like these presaged the rich contribution nursing could make to black America's quest for equality—equality not just in the health sector, but in all avenues of national life. This twofold heritage of leadership and care for community was the cultural foundation that inspired blacks to enter the nursing field during the late nineteenth and early twentieth centuries.

Most black leaders in the nursing field consider Marie Eliza Mahoney to be the founder of professional black nursing in the post–Civil War years. A graduate in 1879 of the New England Hospital for Women and Children in Boston, Mahoney became a tireless proponent of black women entering the nursing profession and having employment opportunities in the wide range of government, private, and charitable institutions that used nursing. She also was pivotal in the founding of the National Association of Colored Graduate Nurses (NACGN). Started in 1908 by Martha Minerva Franklin, the Association focused on the professional advancement and well-being of black nurses, as well as struggled against the discriminatory color bar in the nation's white-controlled nursing establishment.

Another pioneer in black nursing was Adah Belle Samuel Thoms (1870–1943). She was a 1905 graduate of Lincoln Hospital and Home School for Nursing in New York. Like Mahoney, Thoms was an important figure in the organizing of the NACGN. She served as a nurse at St. Agnes Hospital in Raleigh, North Carolina. Thoms presided over the NACGN for seven years. She became an influential advocate for black nurses gaining employment in the American Red Cross, as well as entrance in the U.S. Army Nurse Corps. Her history of black nurses, *The Pathfinders: A History of the Progress of Colored Graduate Nurses* (1929), was the nation's first.

Black nursing schools developed in most large cities with significant black populations. The first black nursing school was established at Spelman College in Atlanta in 1881. Among schools that trained black nurses continuously into the twentieth century, the first wave was led by Provident Hospital (Chicago). It started its nursing school in 1891. That same year, nurse training was initiated at the John A. Andrew Memorial Hospital of Tuskegee Institute, the historically black college in Alabama founded and led by Booker T. Washington. Freedmen's Hospital (Washington, DC) was also among the key hospital facilities that contributed to the growth of the black nursing profession, starting its nurses training school in 1894.

A year later, another important facility for black nurses training opened in Raleigh, North Carolina. This nursing school started in 1895 as part of the St. Agnes' Hospital for Colored People. Two white women activists, a Mrs. A. B. Hunter and Sarah Louise Hunter, led these efforts as the first two heads of the hospital and leading figures in its early nurses training initiative. Together they made this hospital and training school among the best available to blacks throughout the South.

The Hospital and Training School for Nurses in Charleston, South Carolina, was also among the few Southern institutions for the training of black nurses according to scientific standards. In 1896, a local black physician and surgeon, pharmacist, and medical educator, Dr. Alonzo C. McClennan, came up with the idea for the school, and other black colleagues joined him in the effort. Since local city and charitable hospitals refused to train the black nurse students, the first year of the program was simply a lecture course. The Training School planners began auxiliaries throughout Charleston and surrounding towns to raise funds for the program. Through this initial campaign, black doctors and churches throughout Charleston purchased a hospital building in the city, which served as the home for the new Colored Hospital and Training School for Nurses.

One story from the school's opening years illustrates this early health equality impulse. Shortly after the building for the Colored Hospital of Charleston was purchased, the hospital's heads circulated an appeal to the Sunday schools of the city's black churches. The Hospital requested and received financial help that enabled it to replace its wooden beds with iron beds, as well as obtain a supply of mattresses and pillows. Within six years of its founding, most of the costs for the building had been paid off, and some twenty-four nurses had graduated from the school. While the city of Charleston provided annual appropriations to a nursing school in the city's public hospital, this school excluded blacks from entrance. By contrast, black grassroots support was responsible for the initiation of the Training School for Nurses.

Around the same time the Charleston Colored Hospital and Training School opened, similar nursing programs sprouted in other major cities and towns with traditionally large black communities. In New Orleans, black women civic activists started the Phyllis Wheatley Sanitarium and Training School for Colored Nurses. A few years later, these women merged Wheatley with what later became the Flint-Goodridge Hospital of Dillard University, one of the nation's leading historically black colleges. The hospital included a nurse training unit. By 1932, this hospital was a modern, fully accredited one-hundred-bed facility. Others among the nation's earliest black nurse training schools developed in Philadelphia, at Frederick-Douglass Memorial Hospital. Dixie Hospital in Hampton, Virginia, also had a black nursing program that was linked to Hampton Institute.

The superb training and work of black nurses in black medical institutions was not enough to earn openings for them inside the nation's major (or even minor) government and charitable health agencies. Occasionally black nurses did manage to slip through the doors in their profession usually closed by Jim Crow policies and practices. During the Spanish-American War, the U.S. Army hired about eighty black nurses to assist in the battle against yellow fever and typhoid epidemics its troops were facing. These nurses had been employed on the fallacious assumption that, as blacks, they possessed a racial immunity to these twin disease scourges. However, some of these nurses, who worked in Santiago, Cuba, and other foreign settings, succumbed to typhoid fever.

The greatest barrier black nurses faced was finding training slots at hospitals and schools acceptable for registered nurse (RN) credentials. First, the color bar throughout the nation's nursing profession blocked many black aspiring nurses from gaining admission to accredited training schools and credentials required for hospital and agency positions. Second, hiring opportunities were severely restricted for black nurses regardless of their level of formal training. But, third, in their work *within* black communities, black nurses faced another major challenge. Most vexing to their daily work with black patient and community populations was the widely pervasive power of folk health beliefs and practices. Many lay blacks were strongly averse to care provided by formally trained nurses.

In the 1890s, black registered nurse Anna de Costa Banks worked as a superintendent nurse at the Charleston Hospital Training School for Nurses and local public health agencies. Writing about her work experiences, Banks described the resistance to modern medical ideas by the Southern lay black population: "The care of the sick of the South has always been the work of the colored women, called 'mormers' or 'grannies,' but the physicians have begun to realize the need of trained nurses, and will not take any others." Increasingly the black nurses were finding training and employment in black hospitals. However, "[o]ur hospital work is entirely among the poor, ignorant, and superstitious class of colored people of Charleston and its counties— people who are without homes, money and friends, and who believe in all kinds of signs and conjuration." Nurse Banks recalled one patient who said "he will surely die because he took sick on Friday—Friday being considered a very unlucky day for anything to happen." Others came "to us for treatment with such notions as snakes in their legs and frogs in the throats, and if they don't know which it is then they will say that they have been conjured."[14] Black nurses like Banks constantly implored their patients and communities not to give in to the ineffective cures promised by local conjure practitioners.

Black nurses and other black health professionals received high adulation from the black middle-class aspirants and leaders. In the growing Age of Progressivism, strong currents of medical idealism and social philanthropy gripped black civic and professional leaders. Black political and church leaders, as well as business and educational elites, contributed to progressive health and welfare efforts throughout the urban and rural black communities. Prominent figures like W. E. B. Du Bois, Booker T. Washington, Mary Margaret Washington, and Nannie T. Burroughs all believed that blacks would rise as they strengthened their families, homes, schools, and neighborhoods. As Civic Progressives, they were following the inspiration of the likes of Jane Addams, who opened settlement houses throughout the nation's mostly white urban poor communities. Likewise, black women Progressives opened settlement houses in black neighborhoods, such as the Phillis Wheatley House in Chicago, Illinois. These social welfare leaders in black communities warmly embraced black nurses alongside black physicians as the spearhead for racial uplift.

The Civil War and Reconstruction had presented immense challenges to the collective health of black Americans as a whole. The War generated widespread social dislocation and perilous health conditions for America's black populations. The military combat itself resulted in the deaths of forty thousand blacks, an estimated thirty thousand of which were from infectious diseases. In the South, tens of thousands of escaped and abandoned slaves traveled to Union encampments for protection. Under the old system of plantation slavery, miniscule health provisions had been provided to the slaves. However, during the course of War, even this meager plantation care evaporated. Gradually the federal government and charitable organizations took the lead in organizing relief resources and hospital care for black soldiers, and the contraband and abandoned black slave populations. The Freedmen's Bureau, benevolent relief organizations, state Reconstruction governments, and budding black health, religious, and welfare institutions helped to reestablish basically healthy conditions for blacks at the War's end and through the Reconstruction years.

During the decades between the Civil War and the Atlanta University Conference on the Negro Problem in 1906, medical, scientific, and social belief in black mental and physical inferiority was widespread. Nonetheless, the health equality ethos was as strong as ever among the nation's entrepreneurial black physicians, social movements, colleges, and churches. Along with supportive white medical leaders and philanthropists, blacks organized black medical and nurse training schools, as well as scores of small hospitals and local health and social hygiene campaigns. Black medical achievers, especially surgeon Daniel Hale Williams, earned public accolades and philanthropic support for their black medical educational and professional institutions. Gradually, and without fanfare, these black doctors, nurses, welfare relief workers, and healthcare institutions countered the doomsday predictions about the black American race leveled by Southern health authorities and commentators. Black healthcare providers were demonstrating to their communities and philanthropic supporters, if not the wider public, that black health levels advanced as the race's overall living standards and healthcare improved. A public vision that the two races could be equals in both health and in the medical practice fields was coming into view.

Chapter Three

The Black Medical World

Great Migration to New Deal

In 1895, visitors from around the nation gathered at the Cotton States and International Exposition in Atlanta. One of the keynote speakers was the black educator and social activist Booker T. Washington, the founder of the famous black college, Tuskegee Institute. In his speech about the future of black America, Washington implored blacks to pursue practical education and self-reliant communities and institutions. Once blacks achieved economic independence, he urged, the race would obtain political status equal to that of any race or social group in America. Among Washington's most stalwart supporters were the nation's black medical achievers—that is, doctors, nurses, and community health leaders at the forefront of the black healthcare network.

In this chapter, we will see that following Washington's call, over the next few decades black health activists built a steady stream of black-run medical organizations, hospitals, and training programs. We follow new generations of black medical and philanthropic leaders of the early twentieth century, World War I, and the interwar era who devised new paths toward health equality, while making professional advances in the nation's increasingly scientific fields of medicine, surgery, and hospital clinic care. These black healthcare leaders fashioned and pursued a more modern health equality ideal, hammering it out to the general public at a time when the South was in full-fledged Jim Crow segregation.

Between the early 1900s and the 1930s, the major new path toward health equality emerged in the form of black health activists and philanthropists shaping the Black Medical World—that is, a network of medical training avenues, black community health programs, professional organizations, and public health campaigns. This buildup of black-run healthcare resources was a response to the white medical profession's racial exclusionism, as well as the health conditions of blacks associated with the poverty and segregation they faced throughout the sharecropper South. The Black Medical World also grew from the social turbulence that resulted from the Great Migration, in which tens of thousands of blacks journeyed to industrial Northern cities. Once they had established the Black Medical World, the new generations of black health leadership could use it to bridge philanthropic health organizations and federal agencies into black communities. When the Great Depression unfolded, black healthcare leaders and institutions connected foundations and government health initiatives with economically destitute black communities.

At the opening of the twentieth century, a sense of urgency gripped national social leaders and philanthropists involved in black communities. Masses of blacks were living in impoverished sharecropping regions or urban areas of the South. In cities and counties with large black populations, these leaders tallied high levels of infectious diseases as well as maternal and infant mortality among blacks. In 1900, the leading causes of death for the nation were influenza, tuberculosis (TB), pneumonia, and gastrointestinal infections. But death rates for blacks from tuberculosis and these other diseases were significantly higher than those for white populations. Indeed, for blacks tuberculosis consistently ranked among the top causes of mortality until 1940. For white Americans, life expectancy at birth was 47.3 years, while for blacks it was just 33 years. In medical journals and political circles, the "Negro health problem" became a recurrent, if not urgent topic. Although most white public health leaders and health professionals in locales with large black populations were concerned about these problems, they were fatalistic. As a result, they did little to respond to the obvious lack of adequate healthcare resources for these poverty-ridden black communities. Over the next three decades, the concrete response of black leadership and philanthropists was to embrace medical idealism and social progressivism by building black-run medical providers and health programs.

Booker T. Washington was not the only leader calling for improvements for the black community. In the North, after 1905, the key group was the Niagara Movement. Led by the likes of W. E. B. Du Bois and Monroe Trotter, the group emphasized a more activist political strategy than did Washington and his wife, Margaret Murray Washington, by seeking to improve the political status of blacks as well as their poor social conditions. They called for immediate changes, adding to the sense of urgency in the need for equality. In its Declaration of Principles (1905), the Niagara leaders included a focus on health: "We plead for health—for an opportunity to live in decent houses and localities, for a chance to rear our children in physical and moral cleanliness." Washington, concerned that public calls for political equality would only anger whites, worked behind the scenes to achieve his goals and publicly appeared to ask only for economic, not political equality. Seeing Du Bois as a political rival, he also worked behind the scenes to discredit him, forcing many black leaders to choose sides.

Whether in the Washington or the Du Bois camp, black medical and civic leaders were taking on black health problems directly. High on the agenda of black activists were efforts to stave off high rates of tuberculosis and typhoid among blacks, as well as the health problems vexing black mothers and children. Toward this end, in the 1910s, black health practitioners and educators teamed with black social and civic organizations. In particular, the early leaders of the National Medical Association (NMA), along with black community nurses, spearheaded this black health improvement drive.

From its founding in 1895, the NMA membership and activities reflected a broad range of medical occupations. The goal was to form "into one common brotherhood working for the mutual good of themselves and physical good of their people."[1] John A. Kenney, M.D., a key early NMA figure and the head of Tuskegee Institute's hospital and nurse training program, explained, the NMA aimed to "improv[e] the conditions of Negro professional men, and through them, [help] to educate the masses along the line of better health and right living."[2] At its annual national meetings, members read scientific papers and shared information about significant medical and surgical cases and treatments. The conferences also focused on community public health issues, the important work of black women nurses, and practical, not just clinical, concerns of physicians. Public sessions addressed issues such as infant mortality and the causes and prevention of tuberculosis.

As the 1900s wore on, black physicians used the NMA to communicate clinical and pharmaceutical developments, advise on practice issues, and share reports from the dozens of state and local black medical societies. The group also made repeated entreaties to the black nurses community. For example, it appealed to the National Association of Colored Graduate Nurses (NACGN) to hold its conference at the same time and place as the NMA. This would allow members of these two health professions to attend sessions of mutual interest, as well as strengthen professional ties. Furthermore, the NMA's journal, through the 1920s, regularly carried articles and announcements from or about the NACGN and black nurses' matters generally. From its founding in 1908, the NACGN advanced a twofold struggle: first, to improve the professional quality of black nurses; and second, to seek ways to gain educational and employment for black nurses in spite of the discrimination rampant in white nursing institutions. Its early battles and successes came during World War I, when it successfully managed to have about a score of black nurses admitted to the United States Army Nurse Corps.

In the meantime, state and local black medical societies conducted a broad range of health promotion activities in their various locales. For example, in 1910, the North Jersey Medical Society, comprised of New Jersey black physicians, held public health talks in black churches quarterly. Louisiana's black medical society, the Louisiana Medical, Dental, and Pharmaceutical Association, raised funds to start a black tuberculosis hospital. Its physician members also started an anti-tuberculosis league. As in other Southern states, the black Association in Louisiana gave public lectures in black schools, community meetings, and teacher education programs. The state board of health provided a car to the organization members to travel widely throughout the state giving presentations on sanitation and hygiene.

In Alabama, the black state medical society conducted similar community programs. One 1911 meeting addressed tuberculosis before a packed house in one of Selma's largest black churches. Around this same time, the District of Columbia's black medical society, the Medico-Chirurgical Society, had between seventy and eighty members. They helped form an anti-tuberculosis league that drew a membership of nearly two thousand. In Atlanta, six black physicians operated the Fairhaven Infirmary. Under the supervision of physicians, black nurses who had trained at Morris Brown College in Atlanta visited poor households and provided free health assistance.

In Nashville, former NMA copresident Dr. Robert F. Boyd presided over the city's local Anti-Tuberculosis League. This organization held bimonthly public meetings in churches concerning the causes and prevention of tuberculosis. They stressed practices that lessened the spread of tuberculosis—such as adherence to anti-spitting laws and the sanitary handling of food. "Since we began this campaign," Boyd wrote, "many of our people are living in better houses, wear better clothes, and are more careful about the selection and preparation of their food. The churches, school houses, and public buildings are better ventilated and the mortality is lessened."[3]

Black colleges such as Tuskegee and Howard University, as well as black women's clubs, used their various educators and clientele to disseminate health information throughout their respective black communities and national membership base via conferences, courses for community members, and home visits. These institutions raised awareness among the black public about the importance of specific health practices that would benefit both community and personal health. In Virginia, the Hampton Normal and Agricultural Institute, where Booker T. Washington had attended school, held an annual conference on black social conditions. At the conference, black physicians, teachers, and other civic activists came together to discuss black health conditions. The group formed the Colored Anti-Tuberculosis League of Virginia in 1909. That same year, physicians started a TB clinic for blacks in Norfolk, Virginia. A trained nurse supervised the clinic, and along with other nurses whose salaries were paid for by the city, seven black physicians worked at the clinic on a voluntary basis. In 1910 alone, there were nearly 1,700 patient visits to the clinic.

At Tuskegee Institute, Booker T. Washington initiated a "Negro Health" movement. This annual event grew from the annual Tuskegee Negro Conference that brought prominent blacks together from around the country to discuss issues facing the black community and to share research. In the early gatherings, health repeatedly came up as a critical issue. For that reason, Washington initiated a nationwide Health Improvement Week. The coordinating body for this event at Tuskegee provided guidance to local committees to better attack public health ills in their communities. Over the years, the Negro health campaign organized churches, teachers, businesses, farmers, and social workers. Gradually it grew into the National Negro Health Week. Planned and coordinated primarily by NMA doctors, the Negro Health Week organization linked with black civic groups, churches, health leaders, and schools throughout the nation. Major organizers of the Negro health movement included the National Negro Business League, the National Negro Insurance Association, Howard University, and the Julius Rosenwald Fund.

At the same time, black hospitals and sanitariums proliferated throughout black America. While usually focused on serving as facilities for black physicians to perform direct patient care and surgical procedures, each such establishment symbolized and stimulated pride and involvement in community health interests. As physicians graduated from the black medical schools, many started small hospitals in the communities in which they settled. For example, as of 1911, Meharry Medical College graduates owned and controlled six black hospitals in Tennessee, five in Texas, two in Oklahoma, and one in each of the states of Colorado, Georgia, and Missouri. In 1913, John Kenney and Booker T. Washington founded the John A. Andrew Memorial Hospital at Tuskegee Institute, considered the nation's first full-service black-operated hospital. All of these hospitals and sanatoriums were heavily patronized in their various communities around the country.

As the first decade of the twentieth century came to a close, 90 percent of the nation's blacks still lived in the South. The obvious poverty of blacks throughout this region sparked public concern both inside and outside the South. Some of this concern was fueled by self-interest. The nation's medical and public health leaders were increasingly aware of the growing fields of bacteriology and epidemiology that tracked infection routes and showed how close contact could spread many of the country's and world's major diseases. Many whites were worried that nearby poor black communities posed a threat to them as sources for diseases such as tuberculosis and typhoid fever. Public consternation spread even wider in the nation's medical and philanthropic sectors as rural Southern blacks migrated into cities nationwide. Political and residential discrimination against blacks did not equate to protection of the white community from diseases that blacks could harbor. Thus, it was no longer expedient for white political leaders to ignore the health needs of local blacks. Interest increased among local and national political and health leaders in finding public health measures that would improve the health of the nation's blacks. At the same time, the U.S. military was exploring public health and sanitation measures that provided disease-control effectiveness among foreign people of color.

For formally trained blacks in medicine, the desire for improving black public health and physician care derived from both a sense of professional and scientific duty, but also the belief in the positive good the modern hospital entailed for the needy black masses. Ever since the Reconstruction and *Plessy v. Ferguson* decades, blacks in medical fields had built institutions— small hospitals, professional organizations, neighborhood health work, and individual general practices. But now the technical and educational foundations of the nation's medical institutional life were shifting profoundly. Between the 1910s and the mid-1930s, large public and voluntary hospitals became the major hub for providing medical care and health screening. Also, city and rural health bureaus began organizing district systems throughout their respective cities. Together, hospitals and district health centers took on the successive waves of new populations seeking medical care and vaccinations, some of which were now required by law.

The nation's growing international reach in commerce and military engagement also greatly influenced a new organization of medical care delivery. Financed by federal public health agencies, the armed services, and the nation's wealthy industrialists, through their philanthropies like the Rockefeller Foundation, medical institutions developed new medical specialties and facilities to protect U.S. workers and military forces abroad. Diplomatic, corporate, and military leaders made research and sanitation projects to control tropical diseases a priority of the highest order. Moreover, the government had to provide disease protection for the local workers and soldiers it employed in tropical nations like the Philippines, Panama, and Haiti. As the U.S. military and companies fanned out into the tropical areas of the world, medical laboratories at home zealously researched the biology and control of epidemic diseases such as tuberculosis, malaria, yellow fever, and syphilis.

Amid this flurry of research, America's physicians, medical educators, and public health authorities were also encouraged to improve their scientific expertise by the seminal 1910 policy study, the Flexner Report. Sponsored by the Carnegie Foundation, the survey revealed a serious need for medical schools and hospitals to incorporate the growing fields of bacteriology and epidemiology. Although the Report focused on improving medical education, it also influenced all the institutions that intertwined with medical schools—namely hospitals, clinical care, the medical specialties, and nursing.

After the Flexner Report appeared, the nation's academic and medical communities became committed to building scientific methodology and techniques into all levels of the medical care. For example, in post-Flexner medicine, hospital physicians required professionally trained nurses and staffs—while the physical hospital facilities were redesigned to provide sterilized clinical and patient recovery settings. The new modern hospitals also required wider use of newly discovered anesthesia techniques as well as X-ray diagnostics.

In this context of radical change in hospitals and medicine, black medical and social leaders had to contend with two intense pressures at the same time. On the one hand, there were the growing healthcare needs of the black working masses living in Jim Crow conditions. On the other hand, these black healthcare promoters and medical personnel were facing higher and higher clinical and operational standards without the funds or institutional support of America's major industrialists, elite academic institutions, and political leaders. The only alternative left was to try to build a national network of black hospitals, each of which would take on the burden of racial discrimination characteristic of their particular locales. Increasing the supply of black physicians and nurses would be critical for black health advocates and medical leaders, as well.

Booker T. Washington boasted about the growth of black hospitals and infirmaries throughout the South. In 1910, Washington noted in a medical journal article that black physicians were actively establishing hospitals and infirmaries for their black communities. In 1894, there was only one black physician in Alabama. But by 1910, there were one hundred. These black physicians operated six hospitals and infirmaries throughout the state. These black institutions also impacted the black nursing profession. "The rapid rise of the Negro physician . . . and [the] multiplication of these Negro hospitals throughout the South," Washington stated, "has opened a wide field of service to the colored nurse among the members of her own race in the South, as well among the white people."[4]

Still, in the wake of the Flexner Report, most black medical schools rapidly declined. Due to staunch local racial barriers and a lack of teaching and funding resources, these schools were not able to link with the newly modernizing hospitals. Without any hospital training programs to send black interns, black medical schools lost their viability. By 1915, five of the six black medical schools that had been established alongside Howard and Meharry in the 1880s and 1890s closed their doors. The last held out until 1923. Howard and Meharry were left as the sole training sites for black doctors and other medical professionals expressly designed for this purpose.

In the first decade of the twentieth century, rural Southern blacks moved in large numbers into nearby cities like Nashville, Memphis, Atlanta, Birmingham, and Richmond. By 1910, three Southern cities had black populations numbering between 84,000 and 94,000: Baltimore; Washington, DC; and New Orleans. However, as World War I approached, tens of thousands of

Southern blacks began the trek North. Enterprising black doctors and supportive philanthropists hurried to produce healthcare resources for these shifting Southern black communities, as well as for the increasing Northern urban black populations, as well.

The growth of black hospitals increased the demand for black trained nurses. Once educated, whether at black hospitals in the North or the South, these black nurses fanned out to the cities and Southern rural counties as vital leaders in community health programs. For instance, in Chicago in 1911, four of five graduate nurses from Provident Hospital were working in black community service under the auspices of the Visiting Nurses' Association. A fifth was a school nurse in a mostly black public school. Black health workers were proving more effective than their white counterparts in reaching blacks suspected of suffering from illness or disease, and persuading them to go to hospitals, dispensaries, and clinics for screening and treatment.

The more training black nurses received, the greater their value to communities in need of health resources. This was the case no matter how segregated the nurse's city, neighborhood, or rural district. As an example, nurse Lottie R. Johnson graduated from the all-black Frederick Douglass Hospital in Philadelphia. By 1917, she was supervising thirty nurse trainees in North Carolina at the historically black institution St. Augustine University, which operated a school for black nurses at St. Agnes Hospital in Raleigh. These nurses attended to this eighty-five-bed hospital as well as to communities facing dire health conditions. When the influenza epidemic of 1918–1919 broke out, the NMA reported, "The nurses from this school were a solace and a boon to many afflicted and stricken families." They organized and administered an emergency hospital in Raleigh where "the nurses from [St. Augustine] carried on the work for four weeks untiringly and diligently, and as a result many were saved that would have died for want of care."[5] Starting in the pre–World War I years, black nurses worked in community health campaigns supplementing the relatively small office practices of black physicians and small black community hospitals.

During World War I and into the early 1920s, an estimated 1.5 million Southern blacks took part in the Great Migration. Throughout the War years, some five hundred thousand black migrants left the South, and an additional one million during the 1920s. Most black migrants traveled to two destination points: the urban Northeast or the urban Midwest. One major stream of migrants flowed from the southeastern states to northeastern cities like Philadelphia, New York, and Boston. The other route drew blacks from deep South states northward to the large Midwestern cities like Detroit, Chicago, and Milwaukee. By the end of World War I, several major cities had black populations that exceeded one hundred thousand, including Chicago and New York City.

During the Great Migration, the so-called New Negro emerged. Black Americans active in the culture and commerce of cities like New York, Philadelphia, and Chicago possessed a more confident "Negro" and "African" cultural outlook and political militancy. This new wave of black racial consciousness inspired black medical leaders even more with a sense of mission to create health networks to meet the expanding health demands in black urban neighborhoods and commercial districts in the North. Likewise, throughout the South, black medical and community health resources continued to spread into public health roles. Indeed, during the interwar years, the incentive for blacks in medicine to struggle for health equality flourished. It moved rapidly across the black communities nationwide, especially in the urban North, as the New Negro sentiment gripped black America.

With so many poor within their ranks, the migrating blacks had high social expectations, a strong work ethic, and a thirst for education. Indeed, the social aspirations were strong among those who remained behind. In 1865, over nine-tenths of the nation's blacks were illiterate, but by the close of the 1920s, the literacy level had reversed itself—some nine-tenths of blacks could read and write, even if only at a minimal level. An increasingly upwardly mobile, educated black public was anxious to take advantage of the medical services of black hospitals and infirmaries if available. Black doctors were well aware of the potential strength of the black public's demand for black hospital care. Indeed, in 1923, black physicians of the NMA meeting in St. Louis established the all-black National Hospital Association (NHA). The goal of the new hospital organization was to improve the quality of operations within black hospitals for black medical education and clinical care.

Outside Northern urban centers of the Great Migration, back in the rural and city districts of the South, black social organizations continued to plant seeds for the hospitals and medical services that black communities so sorely needed. Black fraternal orders led the way among community organizations that struggled to fill the black hospital service gap. In Mississippi, for example, many white hospitals simply would not admit blacks, and those that did restricted black patients to areas such as basements. By 1931, black fraternal orders had established nine fraternal hospitals throughout the South, located in Florida, Arkansas, and South Carolina.

In Arkansas, black fraternal orders organized four hospitals. With an estimated membership of 70,000 in 1926, individual members paid $15 annually for the health service program. Most notable was the Woodmen of Union in Hot Springs, a one-hundred-bed institution. In 1924, Thomas J. Huddleston, a former member of the Woodmen of Union began organizing a similar fraternal hospital in Yazoo City, Mississippi. A wealthy black man who had large land holdings, Huddleston spearheaded the establishment of the Afro-American Hospital. For three years, he collected an annual fee from hundreds of members to cover the cost of the hospital's construction.

Black hospitals typically provided "lying in" care, meaning they treated the acutely ill or injured. For many if not most black doctors, they were the only medical facility where they could provide in-hospital care as well as formal training programs for medical and nursing students. But these small facilities were hardly sufficient to provide the screening and treatment resources for thousands of local blacks or newly arriving migrants. In general, most blacks were in the economic lower rung and lived in segregated, unhealthy, and poor neighborhoods and rural settings. Thus, they were at greater risk for urban and rural morbidity linked to accidents and unsafe workplaces as well as other preventable health problems. These included respiratory and childhood diseases, as well as "social diseases," especially tuberculosis and syphilis.

During World War I, an estimated 1,400 black physicians answered the call for service. The military had enlisted some 360,000 black soldiers, 200,000 of whom went abroad for combat. Black doctors were essential for maintaining the fighting health and spirit of these troops. Military records show that at least 118 of the black medical recruits treated the all-black 92nd and 93rd Infantry Divisions. These doctors came from a number of black medical schools, with at least 43 trained at Meharry, 22 at Howard, and 1 at Leonard Medical College (Raleigh, North Carolina). Some of the black military doctors cared for black troops in the 368th Infantry Regiment and the 351st Field Artillery stationed at Camp Meade. Trained in rickety barracks at the Officers Training Camp in Des Moines, Iowa, the physicians and medics ended up in France treating soldiers suffering from the gamut of wounds and sicknesses resulting from trench warfare. Once World War I was over, many of these military physicians became leaders within the nation's black medical profession. For example, Louis T. Wright rose to the position of head surgeon at Harlem Hospital; Charles H. Garvin was the first black intern appointed at the Cleveland City Hospital and, later, a longtime civic leader and medical faculty member at Western Research University; and Joseph H. Ward became the chief medical officer of the Veterans Hospital at Tuskegee.

While some black doctors were allowed to serve their country, neither the Army Nurse Corps nor the American Red Cross had black nurses in their ranks until the very end of World War I. With the influenza epidemic of 1918 raging throughout the world, pressure grew for more health workers. In December of 1918, the War Department permitted eighteen black nurses to enter the Nurse Corps. Black nurses worked at Camp Sherman and Camp Grant (both in Ohio) because the influenza epidemic was not simply killing abroad, but was striking down soldiers and medics at U.S. installations as well. Although the bar to black nurses working on the war front overseas was never lifted, at war's end the nation had some 2,000 black nurses anxious to join the workforce. They were ready and willing to take positions at the increasingly businesslike hospitals, as well as at the charitable and public health centers.

At the end of the war, the demand for black health personnel with or without military experience was growing dramatically. By the mid-1920s, public health authorities had two major priorities regarding the health problems of urban blacks in the North and South: attacking the tuberculosis and syphilis threats, and improving child and maternity services. Innumerable cities and counties in the North and South had densely populated black areas. Local public health departments in these areas employed black nurses to work throughout black neighborhoods. By 1931, an estimated 300 black nurses were employed in county and city health departments, and another 179 were employed by private public health nursing agencies.

The predominantly white National Organization of Public Health Nursing drew attention to the budding importance and laudable work ethic of black public health nurses. The following entry describes the work one black nurse completed in one typical Southern county. In just three months, this single nurse conducted:

Inspection of 1,405 schoolchildren
Inspection of 63 preschool-aged children
Home visits to 99 expectant mothers
Group conferences with 51 midwives
Typhoid immunization of 84 children
Home visits to 24 cases of tuberculosis
Home visits to 10 cases of syphilis[6]

These nurses had an immense impact spreading the culture of clinical healthcare.

One of the leading white public health nursing administrators of this period, Dorothy Deming, was a fervent supporter of expanding the employment of black public health nurses. The head of the National Organization for Public Health Nursing and a registered nurse herself, Deming wrote on this issue in the National Urban League's national publication, *Opportunity*, in 1937. She pointed out that it was common knowledge that black health problems in America's rural areas stemmed from poor sanitation, inadequate nutrition, and unhealthy personal habits. However, the public health nurse was the pivotal force who could improve this situation.

According to Deming, the public health nurse usually "comes at a time when there is trouble, she offers service with her hands, she actually does things for people, makes them more comfortable, and shows them better ways of living." By the time the nurse's visit has ended, Deming wrote, "she has won the confidence of the family because she has shown them that she *understands*." For these reasons, Deming and her organization recommended

"Negro nurses should replace white in attending to the needs of their own race."[7] They also favored more training opportunities in the field of public health nursing for blacks, opportunities that were currently far from adequate.

Meanwhile, in major cities, some large city hospitals established separate wards for black patients and black health programs. Frequently these white-run facilities employed black physicians and nurses for these settings. In Philadelphia, a prominent center for the study and treatment of tuberculosis, the Henry Phipps Institute, organized one of the nation's largest TB control programs for blacks. Referred to as the Negro Health Bureau, the Institute boldly incorporated black personnel in its operations. The unit employed ten nurses and twelve doctors. These health personnel conducted examinations and treatment at four separate dispensaries. Finally, in a few cities TB-control clinics were operated on a colorblind basis. In Cleveland, municipal health commissioners organized the city into districts with no color restrictions at its TB-control and child hygiene stations.

One of the white medical heads at Phipps Institute, the prominent researcher Dr. Henry Landis, was impressed by the skill and effectiveness black nurses demonstrated in community health work. Writing in the national *Child Health Bulletin* in 1927, Landis reported that black nurses stimulated an interest in health matters among lay blacks that white nurses simply could not. "Just why this should be so is difficult to understand as there are many white nurses and physicians who have a keen interest and a sympathetic understanding for the negro: nevertheless it is a fact. . . . Where the white nurse fails the colored nurse succeeds."[8]

In some cities, hospitals and medical schools joined together to coordinate piecemeal black public health initiatives. Some of these partnerships organized separate health centers for large black neighborhoods. Local charities or philanthropists also supported public health centers for blacks. These organizations conducted health surveys, and then developed healthcare resources to meet needs that they identified. An example of these approaches to black community health is Shoemaker Health Center, established in 1926 in Cincinnati to serve a community of some seventeen thousand residents. Shoemaker provided a range of healthcare services as well as training opportunities for black medical and nursing personnel, and earned national recognition. Both the city's General Hospital and a large medical school supervised the center's clinical services and cooperated with the hospital. Cincinnati, like other cities, also employed a black physician on its Board of Health, and granted some privileges to black physicians to work in the city's outpatient dispensary.

Despite these overtures to the black community, in states and cities with heavy black populations, the local medical establishments had a clear racial line right down the middle. On one side stood black healthcare institutions and informal black health practices; on the other side, predominantly white hospitals, medical schools, and health agencies. Moreover, leadership at these white medical establishments was largely dismissive of health matters that had high priority among black communities and their health providers.

Overall, in the period between the two world wars, for a significant number of blacks, black hospitals and segregated units within predominantly white hospitals were the only viable source for medical services best delivered in the hospital setting. Indeed, the struggle of black hospitals and medical schools during these years was vital in the social psychology of black Americans. With the memory of slavery and the current trauma of lynch mobs and Jim Crow practices fresh in their minds, black doctors and nurses at black health facilities believed they were ensuring the very survival of their race. Although isolated from the medical and hospital mainstream, black doctors, dentists, hospital superintendents, nurses, and pharmacists were highly cherished public figures in their communities, churches, and social organizations. Their tireless professionalism reflected the New Negro ethos that swelled in the black cultural movement known as the Harlem Renaissance. Working confidently with and among themselves, black health workers served with dedication black communities of every demographic stripe. They personified their race's growing collective consciousness and willingness to strive by means of black self-help.

After World War I, technical modernization began reshaping America's hospitals and medical fields. Following the Flexner Report, hospitals and health centers sought affiliation with medical schools. Together, hospitals and medical schools reorganized their professional, labor, and technical operations to emphasize the biomedical and clinical model of care. These hospitals and academic centers steadily disseminated this core model throughout the larger urban and rural county healthcare landscapes. Physicians, medical researchers, registered nurses, and patients grew increasingly dependent on the hospital's multifaceted clinics. Hospitals became the place for burgeoning numbers of surgical procedures, X-ray exams, infant deliveries, and clinical treatments for acute disease and injuries. At the same time, the general public grew more formally educated and hospital-oriented with each generation. As the demand for hospital care among the public grew, municipal governments, philanthropists, and local charities worked together to enlarge urban hospitals and medical schools, as well to bring modern medical services into rural America.

Between World Wars I and II, black health institutions struggled to keep up with this dramatic transformation. White hospitals received growing flows of public and private funds to aggressively reorganize around the new bioclinical models of care. By contrast, typical black hospitals were small, proprietary facilities that had to rely on their own small community patient supply. Many black hospitals had to open in older, outdated hospital structures abandoned by prior white founders. Thus, these hospitals faced insurmountable problems trying to bring their facilities in line with new technical standards. In the end, of the 112 black hospitals operating in the country in World War II, only about a dozen held accreditation for internships.

At World War II's end, black medical leaders of national prominence like Howard University's W. Montague Cobb, M.D., estimated that black hospitals were providing only a small proportion of the number of hospital beds required by the nation's black population. In any case, black hospital patients were drawn from wage earners and the lower-middle-class "strivers" (as Du Bois called this segment). Consequently, most black hospitals were unable financially to upgrade and enlarge to meet ever more stringent accreditation standards.

Despite the widespread hospital segregation throughout the country, some white philanthropic foundations had strong interest and track records in improving black education, health, and economic conditions, especially by supporting the historically black colleges. Such foundations supported black hospitals and education in this era of Jim Crow medicine. A few of the large white foundations intermittently contributed donations to the largest black voluntary hospitals and their related black medical schools and physician internship programs. Provident Hospital in Chicago, as well as Howard and Meharry Medical Schools, received such support from the Julius Rosenwald Foundation and the General Education Board of the Rockefeller Foundation. Also, the large black hospitals occasionally gained support from local medical schools and larger nearby hospitals to provide training for black medical students or other healthcare personnel. Finally, in a few communities, black self-help organizations provided enough resources for black healthcare institutions to function stably. This was the case with regard to health institutions supported by black fraternal orders. In various cities and counties, the members of these organizations conducted fund drives as well as established patient payment plans. These activities provided a critical and steady economic flow to black hospitals.

Black nurses during the interwar years, like the black nurse community of the late nineteenth century, still depended overwhelmingly on black hospitals and physician groups for training programs and experience needed to obtain their educational and professional expertise. In 1931, the nation had an estimated 20,000 nurses in the public health field, of whom only 549, or less than 3 percent, were black. Almost all of these black public health nurses, as well as the remaining 5,400 or so black nurses in other fields, had been educated at black nursing schools hosted by black hospitals. A few white hospitals, such as Lincoln Hospital in New York, trained a steady, but miniscule number of black nurses. But black nurses educated this way were the exceptions.

With the nation's black doctors, interns, nurses, and many patients alike largely dependent on black hospitals, support from the black community enabled the number of black hospitals to grow from the 1910s through the 1930s, especially in the South. For example, from 1913 to the late 1930s, the number of black hospitals in Georgia increased from nine to thirteen, despite another four closing. In North Carolina, over the same period, black hospitals increased from six to sixteen with just one closure. Inside each of these facilities, struggles for funding, licensing, accreditation for teaching purposes, and developing working links with local professional and municipal hospital authorities were a constant, compounded challenge—mainly because of the academic and technological leap that post-Flexner hospital and clinical standards now placed on hospital facilities and medical schools. By 1928, the South had an estimated one hundred black hospitals, but only five were considered first-rate, full-service institutions.[9]

For most blacks in the Jim Crow South during the interwar years, hospital services or physician care in offices were either geographically out of reach or simply unaffordable. While a small segment of local blacks could afford to pay for treatment from white doctors, many more were indigent. Throughout cities and rural health districts, some white hospitals operated small sections set aside for black patients. But these black wards were usually located in the least desirable areas of the hospital facility, such as basements or crowded "colored wings." Racial segregation pervaded the treatment routines for black patients, as well. In some white Southern hospitals, only white doctors could treat the black patients, even if these patients were restricted to black wings. In some of these cases, black doctors could have their black patients admitted to white hospitals, but they could not treat the patient in the hospital because they did not have staff privileges at the particular white hospital.

In the South, the segregation of patients reinforced the practice of excluding black interns, residents, or registered nursing personnel. Officials of these segregated facilities routinely pointed out to public authorities that their white patients simply refused to receive care alongside black patients. White patients also did not want to be treated by black physicians or other professionals. For this reason, white hospital officials claimed, employing black physicians or interns was not feasible. In the meantime, black patients in these white hospitals frequently experienced staff interaction that was cold or disheartening.

In Northern cities, Southern migrants and local black patients overwhelmed the small black hospitals. Most black city dwellers instead sought care in the large city hospitals. In the municipal hospitals, massive in size and geared to handle charity and emergency cases of all types, blacks competed for healthcare resources with poor European immigrants. Once blacks were admitted into the busy and bustling wards of these public hospitals, their treatment was largely the same as that of white patients.

During the interwar decades, predominantly white hospitals tended to eschew building organized links to nearby lay black communities. Nonetheless, a few major foundations heeded the call from black medical leaders to help with strengthening self-reliant black hospital resources. The Julius Rosenwald Fund, the General Education Board (established by John D. Rockefeller), and the Duke Foundation made improving black community hospitals, health programs for black communities, and black medical education top priorities. The General Education Board, founded in 1903, devoted its efforts to improving higher education and medical schools throughout the nation. Likewise, the Duke Foundation was set up in 1924 with the objective of improving education, health, and community conditions throughout the Carolina region. It worked primarily through the Southern Methodist and Southern Baptist communities. While these foundations were uninterested in challenging segregation in their region or nation's mainstream hospitals, they nonetheless carved out particular niches to facilitate viable separate black medical care institutions. This support of black hospitals even prompted some leaders involved in organizing black hospitals during the 1920s to proclaim that a "Negro Hospital Renaissance" was underway.

Julius Rosenwald, the business leader behind the Sears and Roebuck commercial empire, established the Rosenwald Fund in 1917. Rosenwald believed in ideals quite similar to the pragmatic self-reliance philosophy of major black social leaders like Booker T. Washington and educator Nannie H. Burroughs. In addition to advancing universities, museums, and charities nationwide, the Fund became especially known for its philanthropic programs for Jewish and black Americans. One of its major contributions to black Americans was building public institutions, especially schools and libraries, throughout the poorer black areas of the segregated South. Between 1917 and 1927, the Rosenwald Fund built some five thousand schools, with four thousand libraries for primarily rural, poor black communities in Southern states.

During the late 1920s and 1930s, Rosenwald officials and researchers conducted surveys of black healthcare resources and medical training opportunities. They concluded that local and federal public health and medical authorities were insufficient in addressing community needs. In 1928, the fund decided to expand programs to improve the medical welfare of blacks. Its directors emphasized assisting institutions and agencies that addressed three specific black health menaces: the high rates of syphilis, tuberculosis, and maternal and infant mortality. The Fund looked for ways to combat these menaces by buttressing black medical and welfare leadership and institutions already functioning throughout back communities. Therefore, it assisted a dozen or so of the largest black hospitals to improve their capacity to train and employ black interns, physicians, nurses, and hospital managers. The Rosenwald Fund also provided funds and supervision to local public health departments throughout the South for the employment of black health professionals who served the needy local black populations. Finally, it worked in cooperation with the United States Public Health Service throughout the South in projects investigating tuberculosis and syphilis.

Other foundations involved in black social improvement campaigns provided funds directly to black hospitals, or other nonprofit hospitals that served blacks. They also funded black medical and nurses' training. Between 1925 and 1939, the Duke Foundation gave funds to twenty-two black hospitals in North and South Carolina, including revenues for capital costs at seven of these facilities. The General Education Board donated funds to improve medical education for blacks, including the program at Provident Hospital in Chicago. The Board also became the largest philanthropic contributor to Meharry Medical School in Nashville.

In some cities and rural areas, local, state, and federal governments provided assistance, albeit limited, to a handful of the black hospitals. City governments funded at least two major black municipal hospitals: Kansas City (Missouri) General Hospital No. 2 (Kansas City Colored), and the Homer G. Phillips Hospital in St. Louis. The federal government targeted assistance to Freedmen's Hospital and the hospital at Tuskegee. All of these hospitals were pivotal training sites for black physician specialists and nurses. The federal government religiously funded Freedmen's Hospital, still one of the nation's key black hospitals.

Similar to Freedmen's role in Washington, DC, Provident Hospital in Chicago became a pivotal center for training black physicians and nurses for both Chicago and black communities nationally. At the same time, it also provided sorely need hospital services to Chicago's blacks. As a primarily so-called voluntary hospital (that is, nonprofit and nongovernmental), Provident received its funding from donors and patient services. Governed by a board of trustees comprised of influential whites and blacks, in 1929 Provident became a teaching hospital for the University of Chicago. However, the affiliation with the University required that Provident serve as the training site for the medical school's black interns. Provident also was the only institution in the city in which blacks could receive nurses' training. In 1933, Provident moved into a new building complex. Julius Rosenwald called the institution "the greatest project for the American Negro since Lincoln's Emancipation Proclamation."[10]

Many black medical and civic leaders, both in Chicago and nationally, strongly opposed this citywide segregation that set Provident apart from the area's other hospitals. These black leaders and activists were wedded to the equality ideal with regard to physician training at all levels. In the long run, the Provident intern program proved ineffective, generating only seven black medical student graduates between 1931 and 1938. The General Education Board terminated its funding in 1939. However, with Chicago's black population still increasing by leaps and bounds, the hospital still experienced tremendous growth in the late 1930s. Government provision for hospital care had expanded, and in 1936 there were some 71,000 clinic visits at Provident. By 1938, this number had increased to over 111,000.

In the early 1930s, black medical leaders such as H. M. Green (M.D., Ph.D.), the president of the NHA, had taken on the much more pragmatic outlook that black Americans took on as the Depression set in. While he placed his greatest faith in black-run hospitals, Green stressed that black hospitals could not provide the scale of medical training needed by the nation's black doctors. He lamented the current situation in which hospital care for black Americans was largely segregated and inadequate. It was up to all of the nation's hospitals to make training available for black medical and nursing aspirants. After all, the nation depended on the black medical workers to build up the health of an "unequal people." Green emphasized that for black hospitals, "health is a community interest and the tendency to so regard

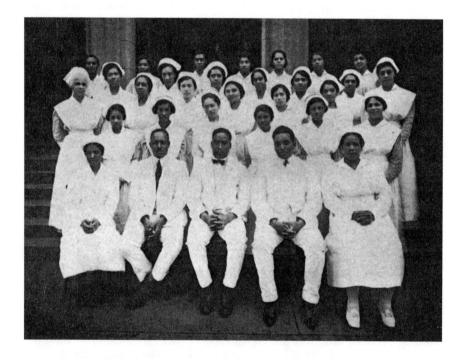

Figure 3.1. Interns and nurses at Provident Hospital and Training School, Chicago, 1922.

Source: Courtesy of National Library of Medicine, accessed September 2, 2017 at https://circulatingnow.nlm.nih.gov/2016/01/14/the-medical-civil-rights-movement-and-access-to-health-care/.

it is the most promising of the changes seen in our hospital program." However, this was not the case with white hospitals. By restricting their services for blacks to just small, segregated units, white hospitals missed "entirely the broader and more useful function of hospitalization—that of preparing physicians of the community for more effectively treating the whole people."[11] The black hospitals not only cared for black patients, but also expanded the training opportunities for black healthcare professionals. These medical workers, in turn, served to lessen disease and illness throughout the black communities in which they eventually served.

Despite the grim domestic and world situation for America during the 1930s, black health leaders involved with black hospitals clung to the hope of establishing a larger number of high-quality black hospitals—institutions that could multiply the supply of black doctors and nurses to the benefit of the broader black community. Indeed, it seems the economic crisis of the 1930s strengthened Green and many of his black professional colleagues' beliefs that black hospitals and community health activism were the only viable future for improving black America's health.

While black hospitals, as well as black medical and nursing professionals, strove to gain an equal footing with their white counterparts, informal black healthcare remained vibrant. During the interwar years, the nation's hospital, medical education, and accreditation bodies were raising the standards for hospital care. Black public health personnel steadfastly promoted these new standards in their work within black urban and rural communities. However, most of the working class of black America living near poverty in the South and urban areas continued to use traditional health practices. They relied on religious and spiritual healing or "therapy" purveyed through churches and folk health practitioners, as well as culturally respected and widely used black midwives.

Religious spiritualism had been the heart of the folk health system during and since the days of slavery. The Afro-Christian core beliefs that had sustained the black abolitionist doctors and healers in the nineteenth century persisted. These beliefs were the foundation rock for the self-promotion of health among blacks undertaking the Great Migration. As Southern migrants resettled in the long-standing black sections of Northern cities, spiritual religiosity grew throughout these new communities.

Many migrants, like many black Americans today, believed that health was part of a total protection provided by God. They saw this protection as all-encompassing and operating throughout a person's daily life, as well as during times of sickness. A letter written by a working-class woman from Georgia resettled in Chicago during World War I shows how her religious faith provided security for her and others in her community in this period of family transition and kept her from dangerous behavior. She arrived in Chicago in time for a great church revival, with over five hundred people joining the church. Even on snowy nights the church was overflowing. She called the event a "Holy Ghost shower. You know I like to have run wild." She closed her letter expecting spiritual protection no matter what came her way: "Well, I guess I have said enough. . . . Pray for me for I am heaven bound. I have made too many rounds to slip now. I know you will pray for prayer is the life of any sensible man or woman."[12]

In Chicago, many of the migrants favored Pentecostal-like worship settings rather than the formalistic services of the large, well-established traditional black churches of the city. Holiness or Spiritualist storefront churches became widely popular, especially throughout Chicago's black working-class communities. Before the start of World War I, there were only a few storefront Pentecostal churches in the city. However, by 1920 there were dozens of such churches. The storefront churches had common features. Most were small with less than fifty or so members. The preacher was the force that held the church together, and membership entailed not just attendance at Sunday services, but daily activities throughout the week. Inspirational sermons and prayer sessions, and special prayers and the laying on of hands, were conducted when church members and their families sought healing from illness, injury, or life stresses. By physically pressing his or her hands on an ill person and praying with the prayerful words of the congregation in the background, the minister and the congregation summoned the Holy Spirit to intervene and eliminate the individual's illness.

Through the mid-1930s, black midwives remained central to maternity care in the largely rural, so-called Black Belt region of the South. The Black Belt was comprised of some two hundred counties geographically and politically strung together that embodied an overall concentration of hundreds of thousands of blacks within the largely rural regions of the deep South. These counties had residential populations that usually were more than one-half black. Rural Black Belt areas such as Greene and Macon Counties in Georgia relied overwhelmingly on the services of midwives. In Greene County there was only 1 physician for every 1,577 people, and a roughly similar ratio in Macon, 1 for every 1,492. These ratios far exceeded the statewide doctor-to-population ratio that was 1 to 1,034.

Although both Macon and Greene had substantial white populations—49 percent of the residents of Greene County were white, as were 30 percent of those of Macon County—virtually all the midwives in both counties were black women. The 32 midwives in Greene County and 26 in Macon delivered half of the babies in these counties. The Department of Health for Georgia estimated that most of the state's 3,344 midwives were black, and they were delivering 42 percent of Georgia's children. Even in places throughout Georgia in which physicians were available to deliver babies, in the poor, rural regions, many women, white and black, used midwives because they were far more affordable than physicians.

The Sheppard-Towner Act (1921) provided federal funds to states to improve maternity and childcare. This set off the gradual process in which state and local governments required midwives to have licenses. At the same time, medical specialties and government increased their unilateral support for physician and in-hospital deliveries. The slow usurpation of the traditional rural midwife, both black and white, practicing in Southern counties or large cities, as well as folk healing practices, gained speed and scale as the modern mass hospital system grew even larger after World War II.

Like the decline of the indigenous midwives, blacks in the South experienced other negative developments stemming from the expansion of race-segregated hospitals and medical science. Eugenics became a forceful current within public health and politics in the interwar United States and other Western nations. Eugenicists believed that legislation combined with the scientific health planning of human reproduction could eliminate populations possessing unwanted traits. Drawing on social Darwinism as their intellectual rationale, the eugenics movement was undergirded by the supremacist ideology that Nordic or Anglo-Saxon people were an inherently superior race. According to this belief, this biological supremacy imparted to the white racial group the natural right to oversee persons considered mentally and physically defective. It also ensured their dominance over people of color, especially Native Americans and African Americans, and even "lesser" European nationalities and immigrant groups newly arriving in America. Some of the most influential works among the eugenicists included lawyer and naturalist Madison Grant's *The Passing of the Great Race* (1916), and historian–political theorist Lothrop Stoddard's *The Rising Tide of Color against White Supremacy* (1920).

As a consequence of the social and political popularity of eugenics, sterilization laws that in effect targeted mentally disabled Americans, blacks, and other minorities flourished throughout most of the United States. By 1937, thirty-two states had enacted involuntary sterilization laws despite the equal protection and due process rights provided by the Constitution. Experts have estimated that some sixty thousand sterilizations were performed during the enforcement of these laws (through the 1970s), with the developmentally disabled, women, and blacks and other racial and gender minorities receiving the brunt of these draconian practices.

The eugenics movement also attracted white medical professionals and researchers, as well as politicians involved with black health programs. Racial medicine had deep roots in the South of both the slavery and the *Plessy* eras. Economic crises in the 1920s and 1930s unmasked serious public health problems among the region's poor. Yet once again, many white health authorities and politicians relied on the idea of black racial susceptibility to explain the high rates of tuberculosis and syphilis in this population.

Indeed, in the 1920s, researchers in the U.S. Public Health Service (USPHS) were anxious to learn more about the biological aspects of syphilis infections and the black population. One such researcher was Dr. Taliaferro Clark, the chief of the USPHS's venereal disease division. Clark played a key role in the initiation of the infamous USPHS project, the Tuskegee Syphilis Study (TSS). Started in 1932, the aim of the "syphilis control demonstration" project was to investigate the effects of untreated syphilis on black males. The project site, Macon County, Alabama, was designed to attract its enrollees from the poor, segregated black communities throughout this county. Researchers chose 399 black males who were already infected with syphilis for the study, and an additional 201 black males who were not infected, to serve as a control group for the project.

The research doctors enticed the men to participate by offering free medical care for minor health problems, free meals on examination days, free transportation for the "treatment" sessions, and survivors' insurance. While the men believed they were being treated for "bad blood," in actuality their physical health was simply being monitored—including through the use of painful spinal taps—for the destructive effects of syphilis infection. By studying the natural course of syphilis infection, the research doctors expected to gain insights into the physiological pathology of the disease. However, for the TSS participants, not only did their health decline, but their intimate partners and offspring were infected with the disease, as well. Even when the penicillin treatment was discovered, the TSS researchers did not offer the participants a choice to leave the study and receive this treatment.

The TSS project became deeply interwoven with the local life and institutions of black Macon. The project carried on for decades with little public notoriety outside of the Alabama locale, as well as clinical medical and government public health circles. From 1932 until 1972, at least twelve research articles tracked the debilitating effects of the untreated syphilis on the men. By 1947, when penicillin and other treatments began to appear, the disease had also spread to the men's wives, some forty, as well as nineteen of the men's children who suffered birth defects from the disease.

While it was white officials who conceived of and sponsored the study, it would have been impossible to sustain the continuous "voluntary" participation of the untreated men, as well as their families' consent, were it not for key local black medical personnel who spurred them on, most notably professionals like Dr. Eugene Dibble, the longtime head of John A. Andrew Memorial Hospital of Tuskegee Institute, a veteran's hospital; and the public health nurse Eunice Rivers. Both were primary in starting and perpetuating the TSS project and, for Nurse Rivers, providing "hands-on care" for the unsuspecting patients.

The roles of the likes of Dibble and Rivers in the project have been widely researched, with interpretations running from innocent do-gooders overwhelmed by the pecuniary and academic needs of their institutions, to willful protagonists. Regardless, Dibble and Rivers, like their white professional peers, had clear knowledge of the nontherapeutic nature of the project, and they systematically withheld this knowledge from the untreated men. Like the physicians of World War II Germany, these professionals collectively rationalized their participation as normal, even ethically sound; merely "good" professional work that, in their minds, was absolutely in concert with their normal personal lives. It was not until the early 1970s that a national scandal was unleashed, attacking the government authorities and medical professionals for their role in the nefarious TSS experiment.

In the 1930s, unlike the USPHS researchers involved in TSS, other segments of the federal government, as well as employers in economic sectors with large concentrations of black workers or consumers, took a keen interest in black health issues. This interest became especially strong as the federal government implemented New Deal initiatives throughout the deep South. In particular, the high numbers of blacks in service-work fields concerned white health authorities and medical leaders, because these service workers came into regular contact with whites. Communicable diseases could and were passing between populations regardless of the political and residential color line common throughout the Jim Crow South.

Meanwhile, owners of large businesses, farming operations, and mines in Southern areas that employed high numbers of blacks also were alarmed about the health problems of blacks. Their main priority was keeping their workers, both black and white, healthy and productive. Finally, business owners with a large black clientele, such as those operating insurance companies and major retail outlets, wanted to develop and maintain positive attitudes among the general public in the various towns, cities, and states in which they operated. They, too, began to advocate for improvements in the health conditions for the black communities within their markets. These converging public health and economic interests led many throughout the South to support the federal government taking measures to strengthen black public health, as well as to increase black public health personnel.

The federal government contributed to the nationwide expansion of the Tuskegee-based Negro Health Week movement. Initially the Negro health campaign had only had a token relationship with the federal Public Health Service. In 1921, the agency started publishing the *Health Week Bulletin* on an annual basis. Six years later, the USPHS began publishing the Negro Health Week movement's annual posters. This partnership strengthened in the 1930s. Following the 1930 White House Conference on Child Health, the USPHS started providing more significant facilities and resources to the Negro Health Week organization.

The head of the federal government's Office of Negro Health Work, Dr. Roscoe C. Brown, also took over the organization of National Negro Health

Week. A few years later, the Negro Health Week organization gained a permanent director and offices. It also issued a quarterly publication, the *National Negro Health News*, along with other community health literature. Each year it distributed some 200,000 copies of the *Negro Health News* and other health promotion literature throughout black communities across the nation. The program became a permanent feature of the U.S. Public Health Service's operations until it was ended in 1950. However, public interest and periodic commemoration of this event by government and community groups has persisted.

Indeed, the New Deal administration contributed greatly toward equalizing the health of black and white Americans, especially in the impoverished South. The various "alphabet agencies" of the New Deal—the WPA, CCC, NYA, and FSA, for example—delivered federal health relief funds and resources directly to hundreds of local communities and millions of working people. In the South especially, New Deal programs and agencies also provided substantial funds directly to local public health structures and distributed nutritious meals from surplus agricultural production. The federal government gave finances directly to Southern county hospitals to expand their operations, which encouraged the employment of black doctors and nurses.

State health boards also received monies from the New Deal federal government to broaden their services. In Southern areas, New Deal funds strengthened TB-control measures and sanitation projects. Other New Deal assistance subsidized nutritious lunches in public schools. The Civilian Conservation Corps (CCC), while initially segregated, put impoverished, potentially troubled youth to work in healthy environments and gave them nutritious meals. The Farm Security Administration (FSA) helped families of tenant farmers directly with low-interest loans and assistance to improve health aspects of their households. These measures led to safer cooking and food canning practices, as well as improving household and farm sanitation. Special group health funds also enabled the rural poor to receive physician and hospital care on a regular basis.

The National Youth Administration (NYA) was designed to prevent high school–level youth from dropping out from school, and to encourage them to obtain vocational training and job success. In states like Alabama, the birthplace of NYA's white liberal head Aubrey Williams, black youth benefited from the NYA's vast health programs. The NYA started residential centers that provided healthcare services to youth enrollees, and attempted to reach broader teenage populations. As of 1940, black male youths comprised 14 percent of the state's NYA male enrollment, and black female youths 20 percent of the program's female enrollment.

The U.S. Public Health Service also took on a greatly expanded role in its funding and authority over state boards of health. The PHS administered most of the Social Security health funds, along with the Children's Bureau. These funds were relatively substantial, and the PHS and its aggressive head, Dr. Thomas Parran, leveraged them to all but require Southern boards to improve such areas as VD-control, as well as the training and employment of black public health nurses. As historian Ed Beardsley has shown, the New Deal health initiatives collectively amounted to the start of the "federal rescue of southern health programs."[13]

While racially biased medical science lay behind the Tuskegee Syphilis Study, by the start of World War II, the idea of racial determinism among the broader medical community—as a tool to rationalize the health problems of black Americans and other minorities—was undergoing a challenge. The belief that inherent racial factors were causing the health of blacks to lag behind that of whites began to wilt, as decades of reports from hospitals, public health clinics, insurance companies, and the military medical services showed otherwise. This empirical data had proven, beyond either skepticism or racist belief, that specific medical care and healthy environments would reduce specific aspects of black-white health disparities. True, some medical authorities continued the search for "Negro blood," or black racial genetic traits, and their alleged biological influence on black disease susceptibility or resistance, with particular attention to tuberculosis and venereal diseases. Nonetheless, as local community health institutions and federal New Deal health programs had demonstrated, resourceful medical care and public health interventions were producing concrete improvements in the health status for blacks, indeed for all Americans.

This sentiment that health equality could be established across the races with improvements in nutrition, living environment, health promotion, and medical care seeped into all corners of the nation's hospitals, health bureaus, local and municipal leadership, and medical schools. Consequently, during the interwar years, urban and rural health facilities gradually added black medical, nursing, and public health personnel to their staffs and programs, albeit in segregated roles and workplaces.

Just as the Nadir period had produced the Achievers in black medicine, the Great Migration, the exuberant Twenties, and the Depression–New Deal Era produced the Builders of the Black Medical World. These black medical leaders and health activists, along with their white philanthropic and political supporters were bent on closing the health gap between blacks and whites. Unfortunately, it would take a global war to finally blast apart the dominant ideas and practices of segregation and inequality pervading American medical institutions on the brink of World War II.

Chapter Four

Civil Rights, Health Rights

For black Americans, the mid-twentieth century would be a time in which the struggle for healthcare improvements took the form of a protracted battle shifting from one place to another. On the eve of World War II, the health of America's black population was generally improving. Yet while progress in black health was reflected in a growing body of health and medical literature, most of the nation's government, policy, and medical leaders focused on only the most shocking black health problems. These authorities and politicians doggedly maintained that the black community was rife with health and psychological problems. This was a central focus of Swedish sociologist Gunnar Myrdal's influential wartime study, *An American Dilemma: The Negro Problem and American Democracy* (1944), which suggested that whether or not it was caused by America's racial caste system, the "Negro community" had become the "pathological form of an American community."[1]

Black health professionals and activists paid little attention to the constant negative criticism their health institutions and black communities received. In fact, America's transformation into a post–World War II welfare state increased expectations and opportunities for black American inroads into postwar American healthcare institutions. A new group of "Battlers" emerged from among black medical and health leaders. From World War II into the 1960s and 1970s, these activists allied with other healthcare progressives. At first they functioned as local groups launching carefully planned attacks against the practices and policies of segregation in local institutions in their specific cities. Gradually these struggles resulted in the growth of black hospital care, as well as opportunities for blacks seeking to enter medical fields.

By the start of World War II, black Americans had undergone a historic upward movement in their health status. No longer a mainly rural, Southern people, blacks were becoming increasingly urban, concentrated especially in the major cities of the industrial North and South. This broad shift in social context spurred many improvements that continued in the next decades. For one, life expectancy for blacks improved substantially. By 1940, the average black life span reached fifty-three years compared to sixty-four for whites. Black life expectancy progressed once again by 1950, with blacks living to sixty-one years on average compared to sixty-nine for whites. Death rates for the nation's children under the age of fifteen also were declining during the World War II years and the 1950s.

Rates of infectious diseases, especially tuberculosis, were declining as a major cause of black mortality. This suggested that more blacks were obtaining higher living standards and that blacks with tuberculosis were gaining more hospital services. Moreover, screening resources for tuberculosis among blacks had improved significantly. It also indicated that black Americans across the generations had had increasing exposure to TB infections. This meant that a growing population of blacks remained healthy when routinely exposed to tuberculosis because of what infectious disease specialists term "acquired and/or natural immunity."

However, the black and white gap remained significant for many treatable diseases, often as a result of poverty or discrimination in healthcare. For example, pulmonary TB death rates were four times higher for blacks than whites in 1960. Communicable childhood diseases such as whooping cough, measles, meningitis, diphtheria, and scarlet fever were twice as frequent among black children. Fatal consequences from these diseases reflected inadequate access to modern medical treatment. As of the late 1950s, the infant death rate for black children was twice the rate for white children, while black maternal mortality for blacks was four times greater than the white rate.

Between 1940 and 1960, blacks also experienced gradual increases in chronic diseases. Most notably, certain heart diseases claimed a growing proportion of blacks. By the early 1940s, blacks were dying at earlier ages from heart disease and cancers of the respiratory system than whites with these diseases. Heart disease deaths linked to hypertension were occurring among blacks at triple the rate of whites. This differential indicated racial disparities in a host of causal factors including diet, family background, gender, blood cholesterol levels, stress, age, and access to medical care.

In the area of mental health, beginning in the 1930s, data on specific mental illnesses within black urban populations had also begun to appear. These studies punched holes in the position widely held among medical authorities that high levels of mental disorders, such as paranoia and psychosis, were endemic to blacks regardless of region or class. Surveys in Chicago (1939) and later Philadelphia (1962) revealed that black populations harbored diverse rates of schizophrenia and other mental illnesses. For example, blacks with higher social status had lower rates of mental disorders than working-class blacks. Such surveys suggested that intraracial differences in social class and exposure to racism had determined the varying rates of specific mental illnesses among blacks in a given city.

Other studies showed that black military personnel under conditions of intense racial discrimination had higher rates of mental disorders, especially paranoid schizophrenia. The pioneering study by Abram Kardiner and Lionel Ovesey, *The Mark of Oppression* (1951), cautioned that medical authorities too casually labeled black patients "paranoid." For blacks "to see hostility in the environment is a normal perception. Hence, we must guard against calling the Negro paranoid when he actually lives in an environment that persecutes him."[2] On the whole, these findings from divergent survey populations and case studies indicated a complex mental health profile for black Americans.

Among the primary factors behind the higher mortality and illness rates experienced by the nation's blacks through the 1940s was inadequate medical care services. This was a problem particularly in the South, where about three-quarters of blacks still resided. Black physicians were the most important source for physician care in the South's black communities. Yet the status and influence of black doctors in the region's medical educational institutions, hospitals, and large specialty societies were exceedingly weak, if not nonexistent. Indeed, the typical World War II–era black doctor still depended on and therefore fully supported the Black Medical World.

The vibrancy of the all-black medical care network we have seen had deep institutional roots. Most black doctors attended the same black medical schools, and then became active in the NMA and their traditional local black health and civic organizations. Likewise with the formally educated black nurses and hospital supervisors. Through the mid-1940s about four-fifths of the nation's black doctors had graduated from Howard or Meharry Medical Schools. Consequently, black physicians bonded smoothly within the local black medical circle or local black hospitals and health agency programs. Fanning out into their particular practice fields in cities and rural districts throughout the nation, black doctors networked with peers who were from the same alma mater and who had had similar academic and training mentors. Indeed, prior to the federal civil rights laws and health insurance programs of the mid-1960s, like black teachers, ministers, and business owners, black doctors and nurses were deeply entwined in local black community life. In the North and West, some black doctors also became important service providers to white immigrants. Even in the South, occasionally black doctors would be in demand from whites seeking medical care because of their skill and affordability, or from an underground cluster of white patients seeking services linked to stigmatized conditions such as pregnancies and venereal disease.

To counter the pressures of institutional discrimination in the medical sector, black physicians during the 1930s and 1940s expanded their public activities and became highly respected "race men" and "race women," as it were. Social surveys of the "Negro professional" by prominent black social scientists during this period, like Charles S. Johnson of Fisk University and the National Urban League, and Monroe Work at Tuskegee Institute, bore out this point. In the practices of black physicians and other professionals in black communities, they emphasized that "Negro physicians . . . get a considerable part of their income from sources other than their practice." Among the many that they surveyed, "[s]everal of them work for Negro insurance companies and benevolent societies. Some have made fortunes in real estate. There are those who own drug stores." In addition, many physicians owned private hospitals, "benefiting from a monopoly arising from segregation in public health service."[3]

Despite esteemed social roles within black communities, black doctors faced professional obstacles from all sides. Public health centers and programs spreading throughout their cities and communities always posed the threat of taking away their paying patients. White employers sent their black employees to public clinics whenever possible, and thereby avoided having their workers use their wages for the private black doctor's health services. Health programs that financed white-controlled medical services for blacks or all citizens regardless of color, also financially jeopardized the small black hospitals or physician group practices. In many communities, white health authorities and medical organizations viewed black physician groups or black-controlled medical facilities as economic competitors. Therefore, these white authorities frequently made it impossible for the black physician to gain eligibility to treat insured patients. Those insured patients who preferred to use a black physician they had encountered initially then would have to switch over to eligible white physicians.

All told, the cumulative and myriad barriers that black medical professionals faced by the start of World War II amounted to a solid wall of exclusion on the part of the nation's hospital and medical school establishment. Between 1910 and 1940, the number of black physicians had barely increased. In 1910, the nation had only 3,409 black physicians and 3,770 in 1930. This amounted to only between 2 and 3 percent of the national supply of physicians in 1910 and in 1930. In 1942, the number of black physicians was stuck at 3,810.

The black nurse workforce was even more sparse. In 1930, the nation's 5,600 black nurses amounted to less than 2 percent of the American nursing force overall. By 1937, the number of black nurses was estimated at 6,000, mostly graduates of the nation's twenty-five or so black nursing schools established for blacks and controlled by their affiliate hospitals. While the overall number of black nurses increased by 1949 (to about 8,000), their proportion within the nation still remained less than 3 percent. The main reason for the low proportion of black nurses was the lack of wider educational and training avenues as well as employment channels. Indeed, this was the same barrier that blacks faced in other medical fields at this time, such as pharmacy and dentistry. Furthermore, public health centers in cities and districts both in the North and South offered only a tiny portion of their personnel positions to blacks in nursing or other skilled health fields.

During the late 1940s and early 1950s, about one-third of Southern hospitals did not admit blacks. Of the remaining Southern hospitals, one-half restricted blacks to separate wards, and only about one in twenty was integrated. Many black patients in segregated wards were indigent. Others were admitted because they were under the care of white physicians. These local black patients were select black community members, in that they could afford the fees of their white physicians. However, in Northern urban areas in general, black patients were allowed in all wards and received treatment similar to the other patients.

As for black-run hospitals, by the start of World War II, their supply was far from adequate for the hospital care needs of millions of black Americans. Still, many of these institutions persisted successfully regardless of the steep walls of segregation in academic medical training and hospital accreditation. Throughout the deep South, some black charitable hospitals and group plans for physician services operated by black fraternal orders had grown strong. By providing affordable and respectful hospital and physician care, these voluntary hospitals filled a need for a variety of black medical providers and blacks in need of hospitalization.

For black physicians, black hospitals provided a facility where they could treat their patients—patients many of these doctors first encountered in their general practices. Few black workers could afford hospital care, and if admitted to a local white hospital, could face harsh or arbitrary treatment at the hands of the white hospital's staff or physicians. By contrast, the black fraternal hospitals provided affordable and respectful services. In 1942, in Mound Bayou, Mississippi, some one hundred miles south of Memphis, a black fraternal order opened Taborian Hospital, with a celebratory crowd of over seven thousand in attendance.

The Knights and Daughters of Tabor had organizational roots that stretched back to the pre–Civil War. By the mid-1940s Tabor local tabernacles and temples had a membership of forty thousand. The Knights and Daughters were formed to "encourage Christianity, education, morality, temperance, the art of governing, self-reliance, and true manhood and womanhood."[4] Taborian Hospital was located in one of the most impoverished counties in America: Bolivar County, Mississippi. For the next twenty-five years, Taborian, along with the Friendship Clinic, another black self-organized health facility, cared for thousands of local and out-of-state black patients. In 1945, for example, over a four-month period, the hospital treated 338 patients. About 50 percent of these patients came from Bolivar County. The remaining patients had come from surrounding counties and as far away as Greensboro, Alabama, and Chicago, Illinois.

Subscribers to the Taborian Hospital plan received a variety of services. For their annual fees, they received outpatient care and up to thirty days of hospital in-patient care. The plan also provided for drugs, X-rays, laboratory tests, and surgery. The fraternal organization held periodic fund drives to raise money for the hospital's operation. The need for healthcare services throughout the black communities in Mississippi Delta counties was severe. Therefore, the county also made an allocation to Taborian for treatment of people who were not members of the fraternal organization. Attracting physicians and other medical specialists from the region's sparse black physician and surgeon supply was near impossible. However, Taborian's leaders managed to establish an affiliation with Meharry Medical College that enabled the hospital to have a constant flow of medical students and instructors in both primary care, surgery, and other specialties.

Throughout the New Deal and World War II years, black hospitals took on increasingly "charitable" and "public hospital" roles, reorganizing to suit the will of their local political powerbrokers, and to provide the best options. Black hospitals remained the hopeful focus of many achievers in the national black medical community. In 1941, Provident Hospital and Nurses Training School held its fifty-year Golden Jubilee Celebration and was still growing. As late as 1945, Provident was Chicago's only hospital specifically operated by blacks and dedicated to serving that city's roughly 270,000 black residents. In Philadelphia, its two black hospitals—Frederick Douglass Memorial Hospital (founded in 1895) and Mercy Hospital (1907)—merged in 1947. The merger healed long-standing divisions between these two institutions and pointed Douglass-Mercy to what then black Philadelphians believed was an optimistic future.

Aside from the fraternal and "public" hospitals, black women's organizations also contributed to black self-help efforts to promote health. From 1935 to 1942 the prominent national black sorority, Alpha Kappa Alpha (AKA), organized and staffed a local, multiservice health project each summer in Holmes County, Mississippi. The area was one of this state's poorest, populated by destitute communities of rural blacks tied to plantation work. Originally intending to provide educational resources to this area, the AKA leadership decided that the egregiously bad health condition of the people would be their primary target for assistance. The project organized medical personnel and staff in local buildings who provided physical exams, child immunizations to prevent diphtheria and smallpox, and other health services to some 2,500 to 4,000 people each summer. Although the project ended in 1942, its cultural influence lasted many years as a symbol of black middle-class chari-

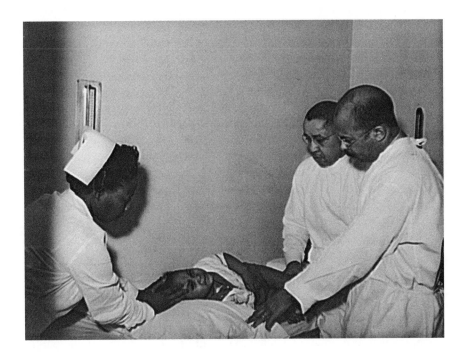

Figure 4.1.   Provident Hospital in Chicago, 1941.

Source: **Farm Security Administration, Library of Congress Prints & Photographs Division, Washington, DC 20540, accessed at http://hdl.loc.gov/loc.pnp/pp.print. Photographer: Russell Lee.**

table medical service among one of black America's neediest populations and locales.

Finally, traditional black midwives, as well as religious and spiritualist healers, were still pervasive in black communities. These women caregivers, along with religious leaders and congregations, remained central promoters of health for multitudes of largely lower-income black Americans, especially throughout the South. However, during the 1930s, state and federal standards and funds for maternity services expanded throughout the South. As measures to increase hospital births among the black poor spread, so did regulations that reduced the scope and number of indigenous midwives. Some states required that midwives must have their clients visit physicians for examinations before their third trimester of pregnancy. A few training programs also started to train accredited midwives in an attempt to professionalize midwifery and bring it under the control of medical authorities. In 1941, Tuskegee Institute started a training program that produced about five graduates annually.

Southern women still had to rely mostly on the network of private physician practices and hospitals for maternity care—a healthcare system that overall remained inadequate for both rural and urban communities. As late as 1949, the majority of black women in Georgia and South Carolina had no physician present for their deliveries. Consequently, despite efforts to regulate midwives from competing with doctors and hospitals, Southerners were still heavily dependent on midwifery, even in the late 1940s and 1950s.

World War II was a flashpoint for desegregation. Initiatives to desegregate hospitals, and then broader movement to desegregate medical education and societies, as well, stemmed largely from the subtle technological and psychological effects of global war. The war marked an explosive growth in the power of Western democratic governments and their technological sectors, medicine included. Responding to the threat of Germany and the Axis powers, the U.S. military and industrial sectors expanded frenetically. Healthcare was necessary, not just to maintain the health of millions of industrial workers producing the nation's military supplies and domestic civilian resources, but also for millions of military personnel mobilized to fight overseas.

Aside from bringing pressure from Allied nations on the United States to back up its international military stature with an enormous military-industrial force, the war also drew the United States into the spotlight of global public opinion. This psychological and political burden required the nation's leaders to face the undemocratic health and employment conditions black American medical professionals and communities were struggling with on a daily basis—not just in the segregated South, but in the so-called liberal North, as well. The Republican Party leader Wendell Wilkie described the pressure this contradiction created when he addressed the annual conference of the NAACP in Los Angeles during July 1942. He pointed out the stark political hypocrisy of American leaders who ignored the rampant racial segregation in the United States: "Today it is becoming increasingly apparent to thoughtful Americans that we cannot fight the forces and ideas of imperialism abroad and maintain a form of imperialism at home." The war had raised the nation's political conscious about this contradiction. As America's efforts in the war intensified, Wilkie remarked, "[t]he defense of our democracy against the forces that threaten it from without has made some of its failures to function at home glaringly apparent. . . . When we talk of freedom and opportunity for all nations the mocking paradoxes in our own society [have] become so clear that they can no longer be ignored."[5]

As soon as the armed services started recruiting medical personnel for World War II, black American healthcare and civil rights reformers began protesting the racial caste system within the nation's health institutions. The nation's black newspapers relentlessly pointed out that black frustrations about racial discrimination at the start of World War II were at a peak. Even blacks who wanted to enlist in the armed service had to "fight for the right to fight." As the war pressed on, the federal government recognized this dissatisfaction. Indeed, the pressures from the war on all of the nation's institutions—from factories producing munitions and domestic goods, to mills producing lumber and building materials—made the federal government and military leadership open to lifting the curtain that segregated the medical service units.

At the start of World War II, black medical professionals and civil rights organizations, especially the NAACP, began battling with federal officials over desegregating the military medical service. The NMA established a special committee to survey the available supply of black medical personnel. The committee then convened a number of meetings with high-level military personnel, including the secretaries of the navy and the army as well as the surgeon general of the army. In February 1943, just over a year into America's participation in the war, the military services agreed to incorporate five hundred black physicians into the military's medical ranks. By the end of the war, there were some six hundred black physicians in the armed forces amounting to about 16 percent of all the black physicians nationwide.

As World War II loomed, the head of the National Association of Colored Graduate Nurses, Mabel K. Staupers, agitated for the inclusion of black nurses into the Army Nurse Corps. Aware of such initiatives, the activist First Lady Eleanor Roosevelt pressured the U.S. Army's highest-ranking medical officer to seek black nurses for the Army Nurse Corps. Integration of black nurses into the Corps finally began, albeit in tiny steps. In the early years of World War II (1941), only 56 black nurses were recruited into the Corps. Two years later, the number of black nurses holding commissions in the Army Nurse Corps reached 183, about one-half of 1 percent of the Corps' overall nursing force.

Although these numbers were exceedingly small, symbolically each black nurse or doctor commissioned raised rousing cheers throughout the black press and public affairs circles. By the winter of 1942–1943, the civil rights leader Roy Wilkins hailed the patriotic service of black nurses, now two hundred in number. Writing in the NAACP's popular *Crisis* magazine, Wilkins excitedly described the social significance of these highly trained young black women nurses. Blacks should celebrate that these nurses "are proudly wearing the uniforms of Army nurses, and bearing with dignity the bars of their rank of first and second lieutenant."[6]

The center for black medical and nursing activity in the armed services was in Station Hospital No. 1 in Fort Huachuca, Arizona. The military used this facility to ready black troops, such as the famed 93rd Infantry Division, for service overseas. Lieutenant Colonel Midian O. Bousfield, M.D. (1885–1948), a prominent physician-leader in the black civil rights circles of Chicago and black America as a whole, headed the hospital. A former head of the Chicago Urban League and president of the NMA (in 1934), Bousfield was the first black colonel in the Army Medical Corps. Ironically, his tenure as head of the black army hospital in Arizona brought him criticism from the NMA. The organization decried the segregated arrangement for black military personnel at Fort Huachuca. They believed the installation was just an extension of the racial discrimination that black people were facing throughout the nation. More specifically, the NMA believed, Fort Huachuca reaffirmed the segregation of black health professionals by Jim Crow hospitals, white medical and nursing schools, as well as the major professional organizations like the AMA and ANA.

Regardless, activities at Fort Huachuca eventually became a source of black American national pride. Over a six-month period in 1942–1943, the number of black nurses at Fort Huachuca grew from just ten to one hundred under the leadership of Lieutenant Susan E. Freeman, former head nurse at Freedmen's Hospital in Washington, DC. Two hospitals with 150 beds each soon were running smoothly, preparing soldiers for duty abroad. Dr. Bousfield's hospital staff included some ten captains and twenty lieutenants. As U.S. troops fanned out across the world to take on Germany, Italy, and Japan, pressure from the NMA resulted in the armed services accepting more black physicians into the medical corps. Black doctors and nurses also served in hospitals with mixed staff, including Camp Livingston, Louisiana, and Fort Bragg, North Carolina.

Nonetheless, black medical leaders still fumed at the discrimination and outright exclusion that the rank-and-file of black doctors and nurses had encountered from the U.S. military. Even though an estimated nine thousand black nurses stood ready to enter the military branches medical corps, at the end of the war only about five hundred black nurses had been permitted into the army, and a mere four into the navy. The editorial headline in the *Crisis* magazine for the February 1945 issue cried out sarcastically, "No Negro Nurses Wanted."

The black medical figures who comprised the Battlers for integration during World War II and the postwar years were likely in the hundreds. Among their core leaders were the distinguished Howard University anatomist W. Montague Cobb; the surgeon Louis T. Wright; the public health physician Paul B. Cornely; the renowned surgeon-hematologist Charles R. Drew; and nurse leader Mabel Keaton Staupers. These professionals first used their own organizations as their base of operation, especially the NMA and NACGN. For example, in 1945 Dr. Emory I. Robinson, president of the NMA, along with representatives from the NAGCN and the all-black newspaper association, the National Negro Publishers Association, began pressuring the Veteran's Administration to end segregation at its health facilities. As of 1947, 24 (all Southern) of the VA's 127 hospitals had separate wards for blacks. Nineteen of these hospitals did not admit blacks at all. By 1954, the

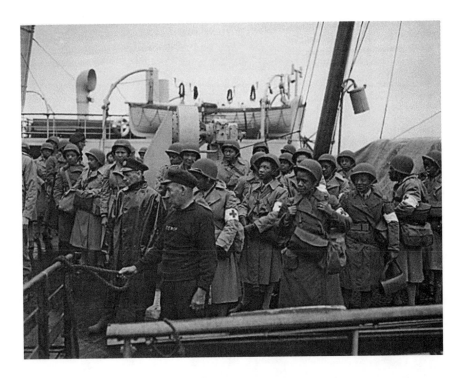

Figure 4.2.   Army nurses preparing to disembark, Greenock, Scotland, August 15, 1944.

Source: **Courtesy of the National Archives Photo Catalog, Department of Defense, Department of the Army. National Archives Identifier 531204, accessed at https:// catalog.archives.gov/id/531204.**

agency ordered the elimination of segregation in admission and treatment at all VA hospitals.

As the military conflict drifted into the past, the black medical Battlers began linking with the large civil rights organizations, especially the NAACP and the National Urban League. In many cities, black medical activists also partnered with reformist white colleagues to struggle at the local level. Together they took on complex personnel and procedural policies to bring more black staff, medical students, and patients within local hospitals, health boards, and specialty societies. Through the early 1960s, local chapters of the AMA-certified doctors' hospital privileges and most of these local chapters were racially restrictive. Undoing these local restrictions took as much pressure from the local medical activists as from the national level.

The political sentiment that segregation at home was harming America's leadership abroad culminated with President Roosevelt enunciating his famous Second Bill of Rights. Introduced in his 1944 State of the Union

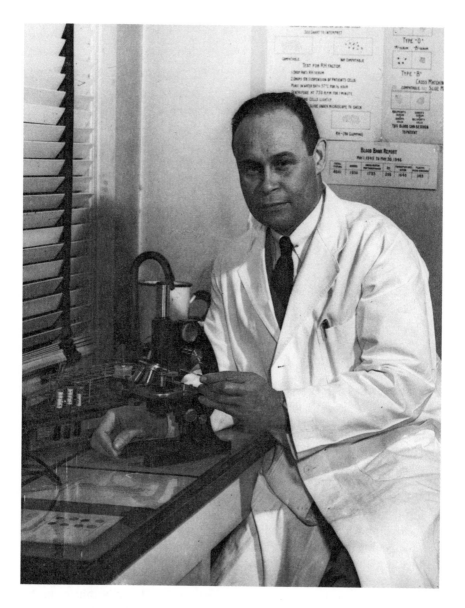

Figure 4.3.   Physician and surgeon Dr. Charles R. Drew in laboratory (ca. 1940–1941).

Source: Courtesy of the National Library of Medicine. Permission granted by Scurlock Studio Records, Archives Center, National Museum of American History, Behring Center, Smithsonian Institution, accessed at https://profiles.nlm.nih.gov/ps/retrieve/ ResourceMetadata/BGBBFF.

address, Roosevelt described the declaration as an expanded concept of "security and prosperity." The doctrine's purpose was much like that of his New Deal initiative: to spread the idea that people in need of jobs, housing, and healthcare could not be expected to be fruitful citizens for democracies. Under this additional Bill of Rights, government, in alliance with business, must aim to facilitate resources that met basic human needs for everyone, "regardless of station, race, or creed." Decent jobs, economic security for the elderly, and the "right to medical care and the opportunity to achieve and enjoy good health" were vital in Roosevelt's new expectations for federal power.[7]

Under the weight of America's highest leaders, the nation's racial caste system, especially as it was practiced in the South, started to tremble as if hit by a modest earthquake. This instability emerged during Roosevelt's administration, but grew more forceful during the Harry S. Truman administration. Both presidents, as well as First Lady Eleanor Roosevelt, championed concrete measures to eliminate racial discrimination in the armed services and other institutions under direct federal control. Starting primarily with the military forces, their desegregation initiatives crept outward to the defense employment and public housing sectors, and finally reached into the nation's Jim Crow medical institutions and hospitals, as well. Government attitudes seemed to be changing rapidly.

During 1946, President Truman faced growing pressure from the leftist side of the Democratic Party, as well as from the NAACP and other civil rights groups. The summer of 1946 had been a particularly bloody one, involving numerous mob attacks against blacks. Civil rights supporters pressured Truman to address the simmering problem of racial discrimination. In response, during the fall of 1946, President Truman convened the President's Committee on Civil Rights. The group consisted of civil rights, labor, business, religious, and education leaders. One year later the Committee issued its report, *To Secure These Rights*. The Committee made dozens of recommendations for the federal government to assume leadership in a national drive to end discrimination. In addition to supporting an antilynching law, the Committee's work led to Truman banning racial discrimination in the armed forces with his historic Executive Order 9981 (1948). Such political measures were the bedrock for the more specific, local struggles that black and white Battlers undertook to advance desegregation in America's healthcare institutions at all levels of their structure and financing.

At the same time that civil rights had moved high on the national federal agenda, so, too, did the issue of access to adequate health. World War II had placed high demands on the health of the American people—whether white, black, Latino, or Asian. They were expected to perform efficiently for the military, as well as work productively for the industries tapped to build the war resources back home. Thus, the question of the adequacy of the nation's hospital bed and medical workforce supply moved to the forefront of the domestic policy agenda. National health insurance provided by the federal government had been a hot political issue since the early years of the FDR administration, and the NAACP advocated the passage of a national health insurance measure. In 1943, the Wagner-Murray-Dingell Bill, calling for compulsory national health insurance paid for by a payroll tax, came before Congress. The bill's supporters included organized labor, liberal doctors, and reformist farmers.

Overall, black doctors supported government assistance for enabling medically needy blacks to obtain physician care. However, many among their ranks opposed national health insurance for the same reason that the AMA did—that is, they believed national health insurance would place the independent doctor's practice under government dictatorship. Major opponents of the bill and national health insurance labeled such measures "socialized medicine." With this strategy, the bill's opponents conveyed their opposition to any form of national health insurance as patriotic resistance to threats posed by communist Russia. Despite the growing sentiment among medical organizations opposing government health insurance, in 1946 the NMA came out in support of the Wagner-Murray-Dingell Bill. However, this bill was never able to pass in Congress, where opposition to any national health insurance plan was more than forceful.

In 1946, recognizing the need for more hospitals, Congress did pass the Hospital Survey and Construction Act, better known as the Hill-Burton Act. The law had been championed by Senators Lister Hill (Alabama) and Harold H. Burton (Ohio), and supported by President Harry Truman. At the time, more than 40 percent of the nation's counties lacked any form of hospital. The law supported modernization of hospitals and building of new ones throughout the nation on a massive scale. Over the next two decades, Hill-Burton funded 9,200 new medical facilities, and added over 416,000 new beds to the nation's health-delivery resources.

The hospital building wave sponsored by Hill-Burton resulted in modern medical care reaching tens of thousands of previously medically needy blacks, as well as other poor and underserved segments, especially in the Southern states. For example, between 1947 and 1952, Hill-Burton funds led to twenty-seven new hospitals in Georgia, seventeen of which served black patients. Although hospitals created and supported with Hill-Burton funds were permitted to practice separate-but-equal policies, black hospitals did receive Hill-Burton funds, mostly to upgrade physical facilities, and even segregated hospital care was still considered a pragmatic improvement in the healthcare resources for blacks overall. In Alabama, for example, the proportion of black infants delivered in hospitals rose from just 24 percent in 1945 to 74 percent by 1960.

In sum, the Hill-Burton program made hospital care increasingly available to America's black citizenry, but it also reinforced hospital segregation. In fact Hill-Burton was the only post–World War II federal program in which allowance for separate-but-equal provisions had been incorporated directly within its measures. As the Truman administration took the reins of federal power, black medical leaders and civil rights activists simmered with criticism of government support of hospital segregation. In 1950, the *Journal of the National Medical Association* started a section titled "Integration Battlefront" that reported the latest developments in their struggle to its readers. Civil rights advocates were furious that the federal government appeared committed to keeping the Jim Crow color line in the nation's growing hospital system.

In the years after the War, the black Battlers found increasing numbers of progressive white healthcare advocates willing to help their cause. These white allies took the lead, initiating surveys and procedural maneuvers to take apart discriminatory practices in hospitals and medical schools. Because many of the white supporters had positions within various health institutions, they were able to work from inside to bring local political bodies into action against hospital and medical school segregation in some of the nation's large cities. These progressive white physicians, many of Jewish background, usually held leftist political leanings and developed skills weaving together organizations and coalitions to attack barriers blocking interracial equality in local hospitals. Besides integrating hospital beds, these groups exposed discriminatory admission policies in medical schools and single-handedly ushered in small numbers of black physicians into official affiliations with previously all-white hospitals in their various cities.

Finally, these activists in the hospital sector began publicizing the poor work conditions of the growing numbers of mostly blue-collar white, immigrant, Latino, and Southern black allied health and service workers, the majority of whom were female. Hospital workers performed a full range of tasks that made high-quality clinical and patient care possible. Allied health workers included nurses' aides responsible for assisting patients in their rooms and wards; X-ray technicians; and orderlies. These people helped patients move throughout the hospital, as well as prepared equipment and supplies in the hospital rooms. Hospital workers also included service personnel who prepared food; cleaned rooms and equipment; and attended to laundry, hospital supplies, and building maintenance. Many allied and service hospital personnel lived in the poorer communities in which the hospitals were located. All of the allied labor segments in the hospitals received low wages and little if any job security.

An important citywide movement to break down discrimination in hospitals developed in Chicago. In 1947, the United States Public Health Service surveyed the health institutions in Cook County and found that city hospitals were racially divided, and that many facilities discriminated against blacks regardless of whether these persons could afford to pay private costs for hospital care. Four years later, an interracial group of medical and public activists formed the Committee to End Discrimination in Chicago Medical Institutions (CEDCMI), and again surveyed local hospitals and healthcare centers that included some sixty-eight hospitals. They found that nearly 50 percent of the city's sick or injured in need of hospital care among the 390,000 black residents used Chicago's large public hospital, Cook County Hospital. At this time, Cook County Hospital was in poor physical condition and facing shortages of nurses and fairly paid interns. Among the hospital's patients, many were middle-class blacks who could afford treatment by their own black doctors at other hospitals. However, because many local hospitals did not allow black doctors to have hospital privileges, even these well-to-do black Chicagoans had to go to Cook County Hospital. Rather than receive the higher quality of care available at a nearby Chicago-area private hospital, which they could afford, because of racial discrimination these upper-income black patients were limited to the overcrowded conditions at Cook County Hospital.

The Committee also found all seven local medical schools had failed to integrate their student bodies. The Committee obtained responses from the deans of these schools pledging to adhere to a future policy of admitting all qualified minority applicants. The Committee also galvanized the Chicago City Council to enact a law prohibiting city hospitals from excluding patients due to race. In its report conclusions, the CEDCMI called for the city's medical institutions to broaden their commitment to equality. The Chicago Committee exclaimed, "What remains is for the people of Chicago to recognize that this is not exclusively a Negro health problem, but a *public* health problem. *It's up to you!*"[8] This group went on to have ordinances passed for both the state of Illinois and the city of Chicago prohibiting denial of care in medical institutions based on race, religion, or nationality.

In other cities, locally inspired black health equality initiatives were emerging as well. Between 1954 and 1956, the Detroit Commission on Community Relations organized the Medical and Hospital Study Committee, composed of local physicians, ministers, and civil rights activists. The team implemented a comprehensive investigation into city medical institutions and their relationship to the local black community. Its survey of the city's forty-seven general hospitals revealed clear patterns of discrimination against blacks throughout Detroit hospitals and medical schools. This discrimination also prevailed throughout the allied healthcare employment sector generally. The Committee found widespread de facto racial discrimination in admissions policies of local medical schools, medical staff appointments, training programs for nurses at the local colleges and hospitals, and hospital utilization throughout the city.

The Detroit Medical Committee excoriated these conditions of racial inequality as unjust. The black underrepresentation through the city's health-care sector clearly contradicted the legal principle of equality in public accommodation. The Committee emphasized that Detroit's large black population was paying public taxes used by both local government hospitals and tax-exempt voluntary hospitals. Its published report emphasized that "[r]acial segregation has no place in present day community hospital operation. . . . The Negro citizen is legally, morally, and financially entitled to equal accommodation and use of hospital facilities, despite custom, practice, or formerly expedient patterns of service."[9] Similar local struggles over discrimination in hospital availability, physician appointments, local medical societies, and medical schools occurred in New York City and Philadelphia. These struggles paved the way for later actions by national organizations and federal agencies against racial discrimination in urban health settings.

During the late 1950s and early 1960s, black medical students and young physicians were caught in the headwinds of discriminatory attitudes by medical school and hospital leaders. Their individual experiences with race prejudice emboldened their desire to see an end to hospital discrimination altogether. James P. Comer was one such medical student working at Freedman's Hospital in Washington, DC, when a seven-year-old black girl was injured in a car accident in nearby Maryland. When she and her mother arrived at a Maryland hospital for attention, they found that the black ward was overflowing, so they had to wait on a porch outside. By the time the child reached Freedmen's Hospital, medical personnel there found the girl was bleeding internally, and despite emergency surgery, the young girl died. Comer went with the intern to tell the mother and experienced another shock. The mother was deeply saddened, Comer wrote, yet she said conclusively, "[t]he Lord knows what's best." Comer became doubly dismayed, by the child's death and now the mother's resignation. "I wanted to scream," he wrote, "that the Lord had nothing to do with it, but I can see that she needed to believe that." To Comer, the child's death "was so wasteful, so unnecessary, so cruel—a little girl died, not because there was no medical services, but because she was black and could not have them. Yes, many white people also receive inadequate or incompetent medical care from time to time—but not because of their race."[10] Comer eventually became a nationally prominent authority on healthy child development and education, specializing in disadvantaged children.

Many other young black physicians were equally frustrated with continuing discrimination. Beginning in 1956, these new Battlers began joining the war-weary traditional ones. These energetic health professionals and activists began a prolonged attack, not just against the discriminatory admission practices of the nation's many Jim Crow hospitals and medical organizations. They also broadened their goals to include equality in the clinical treatment of black patients, as well increased healthcare resources for black and poor communities nationwide.

The equality movement spearheaded by the traditional and new Battlers grew largely outside of the public eye. Since the early 1950s, a televised nation had begun witnessing the onset of highly dramatic civil rights events throughout the deep South. National political anxiety had built up surrounding the U.S. Supreme Court and the *Brown v. Board of Education* decision. After the explosive impact of this decision and into the late 1950s, the newspaper and television networks throughout the nation served as a fire brigade, racing from one dramatic civil rights incident to another. The nation's news media exposed a deeply anxious American public to events like the Montgomery Bus Boycott, and the angry white crowds and National Guardsmen swelling as Central High School of Little Rock, Arkansas, enrolled its first black students.

However, the fight against discrimination in the nation's hospitals, medical schools, and larger healthcare sector did not attract the dramatic national media news coverage that school and voting desegregation did. This struggle in the medical sector for integration took the form of dispersed local events covered by the local press, if at all. Unlike the struggle for equality in education and voting, the struggle for integration in the medical field involved black and progressive white activists pressuring their professional peers sitting on the other side of the racial divide. Health activists usually worked with, or were themselves, officials of local affiliates for major civil rights organizations, especially the NAACP. At the same time, the national offices of these organizations were focused on their nationwide campaigns for public school desegregation and voting rights. However, one health rights movement, Imhotep, bridged into the national civil rights campaign, and managed to gain coverage in the national press.

Each year black medical leaders and civil rights groups had become more agitated with the expansion of segregated medical facilities under the Hill-Burton program. Finally, in 1957, the members of the NMA, the Medico-Chirurgical Society of the District of Columbia (the local Washington, DC, black medical society), the NAACP, and the National Urban League convened the first Imhotep National Conference on Hospital Integration to address this predicament. The conveners chose to name their gathering after the ancient Egyptian "Father of Medicine" and pyramid builder Imhotep. They wanted to convey the idea that dark-skinned people were original contributors to the development of medicine and science. Also, they chose Imhotep because it meant "He who cometh in peace," implying the nonviolent approach the group intended to use.

At its first gathering in Washington, DC, some two hundred delegates attended from twenty-one states, representing many organizations including the NAACP and the National Urban League. The Imhotep group planned the conference as a means to sum up and publicize the inadequate situation blacks throughout the nation faced with regard to hospital discrimination and resources. Each year, it extended invitations to major white-led health organizations, including the AMA and the American Hospital Association, to participate in the conference. For several years, the white organizations declined these invitations, but Imhotep continued to inspire black medical providers to carry on the fight.

By the time of the seventh Imhotep conference in 1963, the movement to desegregate hospitals and take on the more deeply entrenched, complex segregation of medical societies, medical schools, and hospital privileges had gained irreversible momentum. As Dr. W. Montague Cobb stated as the Imhotep chair that year, the group no longer was waiting for the white medical and hospital organizations to show up on their own will. "Their representatives are not here," Cobb exclaimed. But no matter:

> For seven long years we have come in peace. For seven years we have invited them to sit down with us and solve the problem. . . . By their refusal to confer they force action by crisis. And now events have passed beyond them. The initiative offered is no longer theirs to accept.[11]

Later that summer, Dr. Cobb's premonition became reality, as black doctors organized picket lines at the AMA's national convention held in Atlantic City to bring public attention to AMA's racial discriminatory policies. The multiracial group, the Medical Committee for Civil Rights, made up of medical workers, physicians, and nurses, and organized by physician-activist and later prominent LGBT reformer Walter J. Lear, joined the black picketers. Dr. Lear also persuaded the group to serve as medical support workers at the March on Washington. The Medical Civil Rights Committee gave rise a year later to the larger Medical Committee for Human Rights (MCHR). The latter organization provided volunteer medical workers in support of the civil rights activists engaged in the Freedom Summer in Mississippi. The MCHR also continued for several years in the struggle to desegregate medical institutions around the nation.

But at the same time that the Imhotep conferences moved forward, the government continued with the segregated Hill-Burton program. Despite persistent criticism from black medical leaders that Hill-Burton was spreading new forms of hospital segregation, hospital construction and renovation spiraled upward throughout the nation. By 1962, Southern states had built about two thousand new hospitals with these federal funds. Ninety-eight allowed no blacks outright, while the other hospitals continued with separate arrangements for blacks. Many black medical and civil rights leaders viewed the shining new Hill-Burton hospital projects, especially those in the South, as "deluxe" Jim Crow facilities. The broadening of discriminatory hospitals by

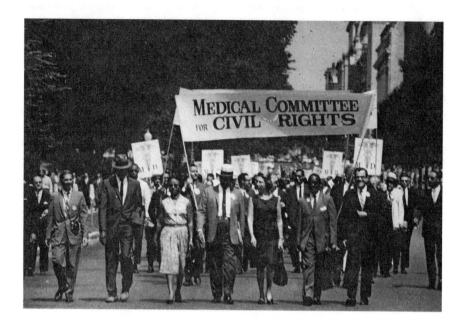

Figure 4.4.   Medical Committee for Civil Rights, precursor to the Medical Committee for Human Rights, at the March on Washington (1963).

Source: Courtesy of the National Library of Medicine.

the Hill-Burton initiative, and the growing frustration among black and civil rights activists about this state of affairs, became clear in a hospital survey conducted in 1960.

That year, the United States Civil Rights Commission, created by the Civil Rights Act of 1957 to collect data on the status of black Americans and the enforcement of civil rights laws throughout the nation, surveyed hundreds of hospitals in thirty-four states. Of the 389 hospitals that responded to the Commission's survey, 175 indicated they had no discriminatory policies, while 60 admitted they excluded blacks and always segregated. Only 2 of the 214 hospitals located in the North that responded to the survey admitted any type of racial segregation. Among the border state hospitals, 3 of 7 admitted to having racial segregation practices. In the South, 85 percent of the responding hospitals reported racial discrimination or segregation as a formal policy.

Judicial battles and a new federal civil rights law soon brought this hospital apartheid to an end. In the early 1960s, the NAACP began legal challenges to eliminate discriminatory hospital practices that were standard throughout the South. In North Carolina, only nine hospitals operated for black Americans, while the others had discriminatory treatment arrangements for blacks. Black physicians were also not admitted for training or staff privileges at the predominantly white hospitals in the state and throughout the South as a whole. In 1962, a group of black doctors and patients, including Dr. George Simkins, filed a federal suit, *Simkins v. Moses Cone*, against two white hospitals for prohibiting black patients. Dr. Simkins, a dentist, was a leading NAACP figure in Greensboro. The white hospitals that had denied accepting one of Dr. Simkins's black patients were recipients of Hill-Burton funds. Consequently, the U.S. Court of Appeals and eventually the U.S. Supreme Court held that in using these federal funds, the North Carolina hospitals had violated both the Fifth and Fourteenth Amendment rights of the black claimants. Furthermore, the resources of the local black hospitals were far inferior to those of the area's defendant white hospitals. So the courts also found that any separate but equal segregationist argument was invalid. The *Simkins* decision brought the judicial doctrine of equality established by *Brown v. Board of Education* into the nation's hospital system.

In the year following the *Simkins* decision, another federal case, *Eaton v. Grubbs*, laid important groundwork to end discriminatory practices in the nation's hospitals. The *Eaton* case involved predominantly white James Walker Memorial Hospital in Wilmington, North Carolina. This voluntary hospital had a separate set of beds in a special wing for black patients. Moreover, local black physicians could not admit their patients to Walker Hospital and instead had to see their patients at a biracial, mostly black-staffed separate hospital. Because Walker received no Hill-Burton funds, its administration argued that the hospital did not have to adhere to federal integration policy. However, the federal courts disagreed, holding that the hospital received sufficient public monies to come under federal antidiscrimination law.

The *Simkins* and *Eaton* cases marked an historic chapter in antidiscrimination health law. Additional struggles against hospital discrimination broke out simultaneously in other parts of the country. These black and multiracial efforts were linked directly to the growing anger in medical and public circles about the poor health of blacks and the lack of adequate medical resources throughout many black city and rural areas.

The reality of black discontent with the medical establishment was reaching medicine's elite circles. In 1964, a leading pediatrician and medical policy specialist, Max Seham, published a study on the problem of racial discrimination in hospitals in the *New England Journal of Medicine*. He noted that death rates for conditions such as pneumonia and influenza, as well as tuberculosis, were from two to three times higher for blacks compared to those of whites. Seham attributed such disparities primarily to the lack of adequate access to hospital care, as hospital intervention had lowered overall death rates for these diseases. In Birmingham, Alabama, for example, about 1,800 hospital beds were available for whites, compared to only 584 for blacks even though blacks comprised about 40 percent of the city's population. In some areas, blacks had next to no access to hospital care. In Augusta, Georgia, a hospital that had been built with Hill-Burton federal funds refused to provide any pediatric and hospital care to blacks.

Atlanta was supposed to be one of the more progressive Southern cities. However, Seham found its hospitals to have substantial patterns of racial discrimination. Only 630 of 4,500 hospitals beds in the city were open to blacks, despite the fact that blacks made up one-half of the city's population. In 1963, the NAACP brought legal suits against Atlanta's large public hospital, Grady Hospital, as well as the Fulton County Medical Society of Atlanta. Both parties settled out of court: Grady gave two black doctors staff privileges, and the medical society allowed membership to several black physicians.

Other forms of racial discrimination in hospitals were as rife in Northern cities as they were in the South. In Omaha, Nebraska, for example, black doctors estimated that three-quarters of the city's hospitals considered the race of patients in their decisions as to whether or not to allow them admission. Although the city's hospitals employed over one thousand registered nurses, only fourteen of these nurses were black. Dr. Seham warned his white colleagues, and the nation as a whole, that "[a]t long last, integration in medicine is on the march. Closing ranks, Negro doctors, dentists, nurses and agencies are grimly determined to secure what is legally and morally their right to first-class professional citizenship." The new Battlers for blacks in medicine were not going to be deterred in their quest for practical equality. "Their impatience today is spiced with anger," Seham wrote. "To those who admonished them to go slowly, not to rock the boat, they replied: 'We are fed up with the service and broken promises. You have had over 100 years to deal with a common problem, and you have failed. How much longer do you expect us to tolerate inaction?'"[12]

Like the Civil War era a century earlier, the impact of World War II sped up the equality agenda for black Americans in healthcare. Years before *Brown v. the Board of Education*, with the rise of Hitler and Mussolini abroad, America took up the leadership of the Free World Movement among its foreign allies. This political commitment to steer national democracies around the world had a forceful influence on U.S. race relations, including public policy toward the health needs of America's black racial minority. Presidents Roosevelt and Truman became advocates for policies to desegregate medical care in the armed services. Their policy measures also aimed to improve the health of the nation's lay black citizenry, including expanding the availability of hospital resources for blacks as well as opportunities for them as healthcare personnel.

When World War II broke out, the Battlers initiated a pivotal "takeoff" phase toward racial health equality that continued through the 1950s and

1960s. They, along with their politically strident allies, publicly exposed the connection between racial discrimination in hospitals, medical societies, and medical employment and training, on the one hand, and the unequal health status of blacks on the other. Likewise, black civil rights organizations— prodded by Battlers of both the older and newer generations, as well as their white allies—struggled simultaneously *against* institutional castelike discrimination and *for* health and medical profession equality for black Americans.

In the meantime, many of the nation's federal leaders and health policy planners came under the sway of World War II democratic idealism. They sensed the urgent importance of addressing the black health equality claim. Demonstrating equality for all Americans in health was a vital aspect of America's claim of entitlement to lead the democratic world. The nation's leaders could not proselytize America as the beacon of global democracy while protecting the racial caste in its social, political, and healthcare institutions at home.

The black healthcare Battler's push against the walls of healthcare segregation in American society began with the racial bar in the U.S. armed forces. Gradually their movement was strengthened by support of progressive white health activists in the major cities. Next, these medical activists began challenging the official authorities and agencies at the helm of the nation's segregated hospitals and leading medical societies. Finally, federal court cases kept the ball of antisegregation rolling. Key cases galvanized federal leadership and agency policies that opened up the healthcare resources of the post–World War II welfare state even more for black Americans across the land.

When Congress passed the monumental Civil Rights Act of 1964, they showed the world that the American government itself was moving toward peacefully integrating its domestic institutions, including its medical care system. For America's political leaders, the choice was either to complete this self-reform, or face the consequences of social turmoil throughout black America. The nation could then risk the breakdown of the welfare-state mission altogether. For the immediate future, black health equality had moved to the center of national domestic priorities.

Chapter Five

War on Poverty and the "Medical Ghetto"

In the mid-1960s, advocacy for health equality strengthened immensely when it joined with the society-wide black freedom struggle. The national civil rights movement, led by the likes of Martin Luther King Jr., Julian Bond, and Fannie Lou Hamer, pushed the federal government forward on political racial equality. In turn, health equality for black Americans and other minorities moved to the top of the nation's domestic agenda. Activist black medical leaders—the Battlers—and their progressive allies had gradually opened the nation's eyes to the segregated healthcare system that millions of black Americans faced. These activists triggered skirmishes in their cities against hospital discrimination and the local shortage of blacks in the medical professions. Gaining the support of national civil rights organizations, they then generated the Imhotep protest meetings, as well as the *Simkins* legal campaign.

The health equality activists also teamed with political supporters in Washington, DC, and major civil rights leaders, as President Lyndon Johnson launched his Great Society domestic program. Johnson summarized the aim of the Great Society initiative, speaking at Ohio University in May of 1964: "It is [to build] a Society where no child will go unfed, and no youngster will go unschooled." Together with the Battlers, the federal government took a two-prong initiative. They wove antidiscriminatory health measures into the Civil Rights Act of 1964 and provided health resources for the black poor as part of the federal War on Poverty. Those involved in health activism also pushed the government to attack some key health problems unique to black Americans, including the infamous Tuskegee Syphilis Study, as well as creating programs to help blacks at risk for or stricken with sickle cell anemia.

Indeed, the government's attention had never been more focused on the health equality ideal than it was in the late 1960s and 1970s. In addition to domestic pressure, with the nation pursuing the Vietnam War, the world spotlight was once again on American democracy, causing rising political interest in health equality and hospital integration. Throughout this process, the Black Medical World began to shrink and transform into a Black Medical Bridge. Black medical practitioners and health leaders became conduits to the predominantly white-controlled major hospitals, medical schools, public health agencies, and community health centers. Equality at the point of entry became more the norm than the exception. In hospitals and medical schools, more blacks, as well as other racial and ethnic minorities, were getting through the doors of hospitals and other medical institutions than ever before. In the meantime, the barrier of inequality became most evident in the racial disparities in the treatment and follow-up resources that blacks experienced.

Overall, black health status improved steadily in the 1960s and 1970s. In 1950, the life expectancy for blacks reached sixty-one; in 1960, sixty-four; and in 1970, sixty-five. The increase in black life expectancy contributed to an increase in the size of the black population overall. From 1940 to 1960, the black population grew nearly 48 percent, from 12.8 million to 18.9 million people.

This improvement, however, was not sufficient to close fundamental gaps in the health of blacks and whites. Between 1950 and 1970, the difference between life expectancy for blacks and whites only changed by one year, from sixty-one and sixty-nine respectively, to sixty-five and seventy-two respectively. The gap between black and white maternal mortality levels remained substantial during the 1950 to 1970 period, as well. In 1950, one in five black mothers died in childbirth, compared to roughly one in eighteen for white women. By 1970, although overall numbers had declined dramatically for black women, black mothers still were four times more likely to die in childbirth than white mothers.

After World War II, improvements in living and work conditions, as well as drug regimens to control the disease, brought national tuberculosis death rates down radically. Yet in South Carolina the death rate for blacks from tuberculosis was still three times higher than the state's white tuberculosis death rate. Black mortality from other health dangers such as sexually transmitted diseases (STDs) and violence remained starkly higher than for whites, which was troubling to health authorities.

During the three decades that followed World War II, chronic diseases, especially heart diseases, cancers, and cerebrovascular diseases, rather than acute illnesses, became the nation's leading causes of death. Mirroring this trend, by the late 1970s, the leading causes of deaths for blacks, aside from homicide and accidents, were heart disease and stroke, cancer, infant mortality, cirrhosis, and diabetes. But black rates for all of these chronic illnesses were substantially higher than those of whites. Meanwhile experts estimated that in the 1960s about 35 to 40 percent of the Southern black population still had not received access to federal antipoverty programs, a factor that significantly affected the quality of their health and ability to afford healthcare.

In the 1950s and early 1960s, concerns about mental health services for blacks had remained in the shadows of national policy debates about mental illness. Under the Johnson and Nixon administrations, however, as financial access to hospital care for blacks improved tremendously, increasing numbers of blacks made use of hospitals for mental services, mainly Veterans Administration medical centers, state and county mental hospitals, nonfederal general hospitals, and private psychiatric hospitals. By the end of the 1970s, blacks comprised close to one-fifth of the hospital admissions for mental services. Nonetheless, as in other areas of medical treatment, inequalities remained. Although blacks were gaining admission to hospitals for mental conditions, their treatment was frequently inadequate compared to white patients, and black resistance to treatment and compliance with doctors' orders in white-staffed institutions was a constant problem.

The problems that blacks encountered in mental health services during the 1960s and beyond had deep historical roots. In the nineteenth century, white social and medical writers who were pro-slavery advocates or racial segregationists had surveyed piecemeal social data and presented studies to persuade the white public that blacks were psychologically more suitable for enslavement or Jim Crow servile status. Following World War I, somewhat more accurate studies of the black mentally ill derived from the reports of specific hospitals and public mental health institutions emerged. Yet the idea that blacks were more susceptible to mental disorders than whites when they experienced social or political disruption, or were averse to treatment for severe mental disorders, was widespread during the post–World War II decades.

By the mid-twentieth century, studies relying on institutional data rather than just anecdotal evidence started to contradict the idea of any specific prevalence of mental disease in blacks. But although these studies and statistics were more accurate than the early portrayals of the black mentally ill, they still rested upon and perpetuated serious interpretive fallacies. Authorities regularly used data on black mental disorders from public mental institutions, where there were predominantly poor and low-income blacks. But based on this small sample, the studies erroneously projected the rates of black mental disorders as reflective of mental illness tendencies for the entire black population.

Stereotypes undergirding an overly narrow range of mental health treatment for blacks persisted widely into the late 1960s and 1970s. During these decades, the nation and federal government were locked into a vigorous national dialogue about the need to improve health and welfare institutions for the mentally ill. With the medical model for mental illness gaining predominance, as well as the rise of wider civil rights for the mentally ill, diverse avenues of psychological treatment and services emerged. Drug treatments, especially Thorazine, and treatments to improve the social confidence and functioning of mental patients such as occupational therapy became more broadly available. Yet the black mentally ill generally did not have access to a wide range of resources. Instead, in the 1960s, as had been typical in the 1950s, resources for blacks with serious mental problems centered on in-patient custody at government hospitals. Consequently, black medical leaders moved black mental illness increasingly to center stage in their efforts to provide broader medically- and community-based mental health services.

A combination of self-agency and social structural changes had helped to improve, if unevenly, the overall health of black America in the 1950s and early 1960s. By and large, the efforts of blacks themselves to obtain better employment and higher incomes had a strong impact. But the Johnson administration created additional federally funded health and hospital resources that benefited the health of millions of black Americans, which the Nixon administration carried on.

In the mid-1960s, a series of national news media stories, magazine articles, and documentaries exposed conditions of hunger and poverty common in many of the nation's poor minority and white, largely Appalachian communities across the land. Malnutrition and poverty led to poor health, and many in these communities had no links to basic healthcare. In a speech to the Medical Committee on Human Rights in 1966, the Reverend Martin Luther King Jr. made his famous remark to the effect that "of all the forms of inequality, injustice in healthcare is the most shocking and inhumane."[1]

Medicare and Medicaid were at the top of the federal initiatives to address these problems. Medicare provided insurance to all Americans sixty-five years old and older, as well as to disabled workers. It financed services such as inpatient hospital care, nursing home care after hospitalization, and ambulatory care. By 1966, some nineteen million Americans already received Medicare. This number rose steadily each year to twenty-six million recipients by 1978. Buttressed by the Civil Rights Act, Medicare required hospitals to desegregate their services in order to receive Medicare funds. With countless millions of federal dollars at stake for hospitals that had practiced racial discrimination for decades, like grass mowed down by a high-powered lawn mower, thousands of these facilities rapidly integrated their services.

Medicaid provided insurance to the low-income and unemployed poor, especially children and families receiving public assistance. While Medicare was administered by the federal government and provided uniform benefits regardless of the enrollee's state of residence, Medicaid was federally subsidized but state administered. Its funds were distributed in line with public-assistance programs, and to receive Medicaid, persons had to meet specific income criteria that varied from state to state. Moreover, each state had the authority to determine the amount of funding it would provide for specific medical care categories and benefits Medicaid enrollees received. By 1972, about 17 million of America's poor were Medicaid enrollees. Although about one-fourth of black Americans still had no health insurance at all, throughout the 1970s and 1980s about one-fifth under the age of sixty-five qualified for Medicaid coverage.

Medicare and Medicaid were passed as amendments to the Social Security system. They provided government health insurance to millions of the nation's most poor and medically needy. Thus, these programs made it possible to distribute huge public tax revenues for federal health insurance into the nation's largely private medical care structure rapidly and expansively. Armed with federal health insurance, many blacks were swept over the discriminatory medical barriers of the past—inequities built on racial exclusion and unaffordable costs for services. However, these new health insurance programs were not sufficient to nail medical care inequality in its coffin over the long haul. For example, private physicians and hospitals preferred not to treat Medicaid recipients. Medicaid reimbursements to these caregivers were significantly lower than payments from privately insured or middle-class paying patients. This practice resulted in many Medicaid recipients of poor, minority communities lacking sufficient funds for access to a wide range of local hospitals.

Federal antipoverty and nutrition programs, Medicare and Medicaid, children's development programs like Head Start, and other federal community health resources did bring about material improvements to blacks' legal, economic, and social conditions. Generations before, these blacks would have been living and dying in poverty. The improvements enabled a growing black working- and middle-class to acquire safer and healthier housing stock, food and clothing, workplace conditions, and municipal and agricultural environments.

Nonetheless, despite gains from the Civil Rights Movement, many African Americans still saw little improvement in their overall lives, especially in urban areas. While the federal government unleashed its civil rights and health reform programs, scores of cities were experiencing race riots. In 1964, riots flared in Rochester (New York), Philadelphia, and other cities, and in each following year, dozens more occurred in other cities. In 1967, with the national political climate deeply troubled over race relations, President Johnson convened the National Advisory Committee on Civil Disorders or the so-called Kerner Commission. The final report of the commission affirmed that racial discrimination and poverty were the primary causes for the riots and gained headline coverage across the nation. Its central, blistering finding echoed throughout America's popular media: The nation was splitting apart along the color line: "Our nation is moving toward two societies, one black, one white—separate and unequal."

The Kerner Commission recommended that all levels of government develop reforms in housing, education, and social services to improve the lives of black Americans. The Reverend Martin Luther King Jr. called the report a "physician's warning of approaching death, with a prescription for life. The duty of every American is to administer the remedy without regard for the cost and without delay."[2] As fate would have it, Reverend King's assassination in 1968 fanned the flames of even more urban riots. The nation expected the president and Congress to respond, and each year, from 1964 through the early 1970s, it did with new health reform legislation and resources.

As government and health authorities implemented antipoverty and community health programs, in city after city they encountered harsh realities. Health commentators and much of the public used the term "medical ghetto" to describe the acute gaps in healthcare delivery these impoverished urban and rural black communities routinely faced. At the center of the situation was the lack of coherent long-term care organized by primary-care physicians or local hospitals providing clinical specialty medicine. The residents of the urban poor areas received medical care from two primary sources: emergency rooms and outpatient services at often overburdened public hospitals; or small office or "solo" practices of private physicians, mostly black. Doctor's visits amounted to about 60 percent of this care, while hospital outpatient services some 20 percent. Small community facilities like health centers provided just 1 percent. The medical ghetto existed in every major black community.

For blacks living in city ghettos and poor rural areas, the tangle of fragmented healthcare resources hardly met their medical needs. In 1960, the black doctor–to–black population ratio nationally was 1 to 5,000 compared to the national average ratio of 1 doctor for every 670 persons. Compared to middle-class and suburban communities, the supply of solo-practice physicians for heavily populated, low-income black and minority city sections and rural areas was woefully small. In the South, the black doctor–to–black population ratios was 1 per 6,203 in the thirteen southern states. In South Carolina and Mississippi, the black physician-to-black population ratio was 1 to 12,561 and 1 to 18,132 respectively.

Throughout the nation's major cities, areas with high concentrations of black residents, such as the Watts section of Los Angeles, in which the famous 1965 "long hot summer" riot occurred, only 106 doctors were serving some 252,000 residents. This amounted to a doctor-to-resident ratio of 1 to 2,377. In the core of Baltimore City, which was heavily populated with black residents, in 1969 there were only 100 physicians practicing amid an estimated population of 300,000, amounting to a doctor-patient ratio of 1 for every 3,000 persons. That same year, in the black "ghetto" area of Boston comprised of some 80,000 residents, only fifty physicians were in practice: a ratio of 1 to every 1,600 residents.

Physicians and nurses working in ghetto health facilities or solo physician offices faced heavy patient loads and troubled neighborhood conditions. They linked their situations directly to societal racism. John L. S. Holloman Jr., a black physician and head of the Physician's Forum, described the challenges. Addressing a national conference on "Medicine in the Ghetto" in 1969, he remarked: "The ghetto physician is in the first line of defense against the [constant] onslaught of disability and disease." Holloman pointed out that the ill-health rampant in the "ghetto stands as a monument to our national failure. It is ugly, dirty, diseased, and decaying. It symbolizes the moribund city." He warned that these conditions could grow in the future: "The problems of the ghetto dweller are an integral component of the larger catastrophe of our cities."[3]

There were many university affiliated/teaching hospitals located in or near the poor, mostly black neighborhoods in major cities that served as urban hubs for biomedical research and clinical specialties. However, these facilities were not organized to provide the long-term primary care local communities needed. As one policy study stated in 1971, these "[m]ajor centers of medical research and education . . . abut on urban slums, which are some of the nation's most disgraceful backwaters of medical neglect."[4] While the hospitals did provide emergency room care, usually these emergency units were unprepared to handle the scope of medical conditions that characterized incoming patients. Emergency rooms in urban public hospitals that served the ghettos were routinely packed with people who would be better served by primary-care physicians' offices.

Another term that gained popularity in municipal, political, and health activist circles at this time was the "ghetto hospital." Ghetto hospitals were largely the older municipal or public general hospitals that had emerged during the Civil War through World War I to provide care for the indigent sick. These hospitals still, compared to other hospitals in their city, cared for a large percentage of the nearby poor. In major cities, some of the voluntary hospitals, including the relatively tiny number of black hospitals, made up a subset of the ghetto hospitals. Usually locally administered by nonprofit bodies like religious denominations and philanthropies, and funded by voluntary contributions and paying patients, these hospitals provided care primarily in impoverished black and Hispanic neighborhoods. Medical ghetto hospitals also were worksites for the growing labor segment of black and Hispanic allied health workers, who usually lived in the communities these hospitals served.

Decades of underfunding left many public general hospitals in poor physical condition and insufficiently staffed to perform the wide range of medical services surrounding communities needed. Academic affiliation proved to be the fiscal and operational salvation for many public hospitals. However, as was the case with most of the black hospitals just before World War II, urban public and voluntary hospitals were under constant pressure not to sink financially. They had little or no influence in the streams of public and private insurance funds flowing into the wealthier, academically accredited major hospitals. Thus, the hospitals in black neighborhoods, whether deemed a ghetto hospital or not, had insufficient financial resources to meet the vast demands from the urban poor and minority populations.

In response to the growing national and black community dissatisfaction with medical ghetto conditions, the federal government and health philanthropists responded on a massive scale. The government funded community health resources throughout many of the nation's most poor urban and rural communities. Beginning with the War on Poverty, and then continuing under President Nixon, a wave of community health centers opened their doors in impoverished neighborhoods and rural areas.

Starting in 1966, Senator Edward Kennedy of Massachusetts led Congress in the federal government initiatives to eliminate the medical ghetto for the nation's urban and rural poor by heading the drive for federal programs to start community health centers. These multiservice facilities targeted major cities and rural areas with large black, white, and ethnic poor populations. Established under the U.S. Office of Equal Opportunity (OEO), the centers harkened back to the neighborhood health centers of the early twentieth century. The OEO planned the health centers for easy accessibility for neighborhood residents who normally were unable to travel to healthcare facilities. Each center designed its services to meet the medical needs of the surrounding neighborhoods. In addition to providing primary care, the centers also served as referral sites that screened and referred residents to the city's larger, more specialized hospitals and clinics. Another feature of the centers was their governance structure, which included civic leaders from the community the facility served.

Over the next five years, OEO established some 150 centers and projects, two-thirds of which offered comprehensive health services. In the first few years, hospitals administered about one-half of these centers, medical schools about two-fifths, and health departments about one-tenth. However, strong pressure from black and minority communities to more fully participate in the planning and operations of these centers changed this pattern. By 1971, community and health provider partnerships—some called health corporations—ran one-half of the centers, hospitals only operated about one-tenth, and medical schools ran even fewer.

Another government program that increased healthcare resources for the urban poor was the Model Cities program, officially part of the Demonstration Cities and Metropolitan Development Act (1966). President Johnson placed Robert Weaver, the new secretary of Housing and Urban Development (HUD) and the nation's first black American cabinet member, in charge of this program. By 1973, the program was providing government subsidies for health services and neighborhood health centers in 115 communities throughout the country. These communities had substantial populations of poor blacks, whites, and other ethnic groups.

While the community health centers of the late 1960s and early 1970s seemed similar to the neighborhood health centers and hygiene campaigns of the early twentieth century, these new centers were administered by government, hospital, and/or medical school authorities, and funded directly with federal revenue. Community health centers also became training grounds for local residents who gained employment in these facilities. Many of these workers later became employees in allied health work in their city's growing healthcare sector.

Many private groups also started free clinics throughout poor urban communities to combat the inadequate, ghetto healthcare situation. Prominent among such local centers were the Black Panther Party's free clinics. The organizers of the Black Panther centers had been influenced by the health ideas of charismatic international revolutionaries, including the anticolonial, Martiniquian psychiatrist Franz Fanon; the Cuban guerilla fighter Ernesto "Che" Guevara; and Chinese leader Mao Tse-tung (pinyin: Mao Zedong). All of these figures stressed popular health campaigns and the mobilization of health workers to provide primary healthcare, promote grassroots health education, and improve environmental conditions. Mao himself had promoted the massive "barefoot doctor" campaign as a key part of the Chinese Revolution.

Free health clinics and sickle cell programs cropped up in black communities in several cities. Usually run by a handful of part-time staff, they offered free exams and some primary services, as well as promoted neighborhood and public awareness of health hazards like sickle cell disease, which threatened residents of poor communities. Because these clinics were voluntary and were miniscule in size and number, they were not comparable to the traditional black hospitals. Instead, they personified the growing black consciousness and militant defensiveness burning widely in black working-class communities at this time. Progressive activists among women and other minorities, especially Latino Americans, Native Americans, and Asian Americans, started free clinics and health promotion activities for their particular communities, as well. Each group focused on their own health priorities and community-based solutions through local health centers, as well as grassroots health campaigns.

During this period of political turbulence, discrimination in mental health services continued. When urban riots broke out across the nation, many white staff in mental health services at hospitals and agencies were averse to treating mentally ill black patients. This "informal" discrimination was also reflected in the treatment blacks received if admitted into the hospital setting. Black patients were frequently misdiagnosed, especially if aggressive behavior was one of the symptoms. For example, studies found that black patients were often diagnosed with paranoid schizophrenia when actually they were manic-depressive, resulting in these patients receiving inappropriate drug regimens. Discrimination in the mental health field complemented the social psychological fear that took hold of much of the white public as they witnessed urban black riots either in their own cities or in the national media. Indeed, social fear of a peculiar aggressiveness of black urban residents was a driving force behind the mass "white flight" or suburbanization that occurred during the 1960s and 1970s.

A new generation of Battlers emerged among black psychiatrists and other mental health professionals. They viewed black mental illness in fundamentally different ways compared to mainstream mental health authorities. These professionals criticized the limited range of services and treatment expectations for blacks in their communities and cities. They accused the mainstream psychiatry profession of overlooking the extreme psychological trepidation that racism caused blacks. As one psychiatrist among these activist professionals emphasized, black Americans of all social backgrounds faced a common environment of racism. This racism posed mental and material hurdles every black had to clear individually. All blacks are potentially "psychologically terrorized, politically tyrannized, social minimized and economically ignored."[5] Routine diagnoses and treatments that ignored this factor, in the end, were destined to be ineffective.

Black psychologists offered field studies and personal accounts of experiences with black patients to expose discrimination in all phases of mental health services. These materials confirmed that if blacks throughout the nation were exhibiting mental problems at disproportionately higher rates compared to whites, it was merely an adaptation to widespread white aggression. According to black psychiatrists, aggression or rage among blacks was not a form of psychopathology. It was neither inexplicable nor some highly personal form of mental derangement in its origins. Instead mental states in blacks involving moods—for example, anger or phobias—were predictable responses to intolerable racism.

The book *Black Rage* (1969) by black psychiatrists William H. Grier and Price M. Cobbs was a militant tract against white psychiatry, which attracted a national audience across the color line. *Black Rage* intended to obliterate the stereotype that the black mentally ill were writhing with inane aggression. Grier and Cobbs explained in simple language the overbearing racism pervading the "white" social world in which blacks had to function. Facing an environment of constant social degradation and powerlessness, black men and women possessed a rather logical "cultural paranoia." Blacks had no choice but to contest whites in order to survive. "If blacks are frightened . . .

consider what frightens them and consider what happens when they feel cornered," they wrote. Further, this rage surfaced "when there is no further lie one can believe, when one finally sees he is permanently cast as a victim, and when finally the sleeping giant wakes and turns upon his tormentors."[6]

Progressive black and white psychologists also offered case studies and surveys that cracked the pervasive stereotype that blacks did not experience certain mental disorders due to inborn racial characteristics. Public mental health institutions tended to have a higher proportion of black patients, thus fueling the notion that blacks as a whole have higher rates of mental illness compared to whites. However, these newer studies indicated that while various types of psychopathologies—for example, anxiety, phobias, or depression—did, indeed, occur at significant levels among blacks, these mental illnesses prevailed within black populations at rates generally comparable to whites of similar socioeconomic status, gender, and age. Finally, while early surveys showed that blacks had higher rates of certain psychological ailments like phobic disorders, the newer research showed that overconcentration of poverty, other social stressors, and discriminatory admission (or exclusion) practices at mental institutions could explain these disparities.

In the decade that followed the Community Mental Health Centers Construction Act of 1963, deinstitutionalization of the mentally ill spread nationally. The central purpose of the law was to drastically reduce mental health patients in custodial institutions. Instead, patients were to receive more individualized treatment in community settings. The law supported the policy that would open an estimated two thousand community-based centers to treat the mentally ill. Local hospitals and regional bodies would coordinate a wide range of ambulatory psychological services. Compared to the early 1960s, by the early 1970s substantially larger numbers of mentally ill blacks were receiving outpatient treatment in regional mental health centers. Still, even at these community mental health centers, blacks most frequently received the lowest level of treatment, often rendered by nonprofessional staff. In fact, these facilities rarely employed black professional staff who could have likely given more accurate diagnoses and treatment for black patients.

Some mental health specialists suggested that blackness could be a source of psychological strength. These psychiatrists and social scientists stressed that black culture was a source of coalition building and resilience despite the debilitating psychological pressure of racism and physical illnesses. These qualities had manifested going back to the Yellow Fever Epidemic of 1787, the National Negro Health Weeks of the Great Migration and World War II decades, and other black social welfare and health education programs throughout the centuries. Indeed, a new group of black health professionals, the black medical Bridge Builders, who were aware of their history, culture, and community's resilient qualities, took the lead in their various staff and advisory capacities at predominantly white institutions. These black health workers tried to build new healthcare delivery models—models that incorporated black community self-help approaches as well as resilient household and neighborhood practices.

For example, parenting styles in traditional black households had successfully prevented black youngsters from adopting the habit of smoking. Epidemiologists in the 1960s and 1970s discovered that compared to white and Latino youth, black youth acquired smoking habits far less frequently. Smoking had been rising on the nation's health agenda as a most serious cause of preventable diseases, disability, and mortality. These health problems included several forms of cancers, heart disease and stroke, respiratory diseases, and pregnancy complications. This protective "informal" cultural capital—practices and beliefs within families, churches, communities, and other intimate associations—made up for deficiencies in preventive healthcare and formal psychological services.

The Civil Rights Act, Medicaid and Medicare, and federal court decisions had led to the rapid integration of thousands of the nation's hospitals and health agencies receiving federal funds. Likewise labor and political movements had forced government to bar segregation in employment involving federal contracts. By the mid-1960s, the federal government was poised to require "affirmative action" policies in education and employment. The combination of more hospitals and more federal government oversight of integration created a strong market for black medical professionals and allied health employees. They were sought not only for their skills, but also for their ability to serve as a bridge to local communities of color. These black healthcare workers would essentially serve the vast new black patient-consumer market for America's hospital and medical school establishment. Ultimately, the entire spectrum of the nation's health profession schools and professional specialties found it desirable to end the tradition of racial exclusion.

Beginning in the mid-1960s, predominantly white medical and dental schools began intensive efforts to increase black enrollment. They designed affirmative action programs to recruit and graduate significant numbers of black and racial minority medical students. The federal government played a major role. Congress provided more support for manpower training programs and expanded educational assistance funds to improve the quantity and distribution of minority physicians and other health professionals. Moreover, foundations joined in to develop innovative means to support these integration efforts. The Macy Foundation, Rockefeller Foundation, Robert Wood Johnson Foundation, and the National Medical Fellowships, among others, established programs to increase the pool of black and minority students applying to and completing medical schools. They also supplied funds to strengthen premed education at HBCUs, mentorship programs before and during medical school, and scholarships. For example, the Robert Wood Johnson Foundation provided funds for mentoring programs and scholarships. In 1970, the Association of American Medical Schools headed a task force on increasing minority enrollment with representatives from the nation's largest health organizations, including the AMA, the American Hospital Association, and the NMA. It set a goal of 12 percent minority student enrollment by 1973 in the nation's medical schools—roughly the proportion of the nation's population that was black.

The combination of government affirmative action and philanthropic programs, along with a focused national commitment from the nation's medical schools, had a historic impact. It sped the entry of blacks into the medical school–to–doctor pipeline at a frenetic rate. In the 1968–1969 academic year, only 783, or 2.2 percent, of the nation's medical students were black. This number rose to 1,042 in 1969–1970. By 1975, black medical school enrollment reached 3,456, or about 7.5 percent of the total medical students nationwide. From that point on, the percentage leveled off and remained at about 6 percent through the 1980s.

Incorporating black physicians, nurses, and other health workers into new roles as champions of integration was not a smooth process. In many instances, blacks working with white peers experienced culture shock. Black professionals also often witnessed white racism firsthand. Dr. James Comer, M.D., a child psychiatrist later prominent in his field, was constantly troubled by the arrogant attitudes of white colleagues. As a new medical school graduate in the 1960s, Comer worked at a municipal health clinic in Washington, DC. Many patients at the clinic were elderly blue-collar workers, who had worked throughout their entire lives for survival wages. Some were now on public welfare. Yet, to one white colleague at the clinic, these patients, and all black welfare recipients coming to the clinic, were merely "taking a free ride."

Actually, Comer observed, many of the black working poor continued doing their jobs even though they had obvious health problems. He knew of one elderly black clinic aide who could not afford to stop working even while she was dying of cancer. Comer developed a theory to explain to himself the cynical attitudes of his white professional peers: "I now understand the phenomenon not as mental illness, but as a kind of collective defect in the national ego and superego; a blind spot that permits otherwise intelligent people to see, think and act in a racist way without the expected level of guilt and pain." He called this collective attitude a kind of "white mind."[7]

The traditional Black Medical World paid a high price for integration. Through 1950, the majority (an estimated 85 percent) of black medical students graduated from the nation's two black medical schools, Howard and Meharry. However, as the recruitment by predominantly white medical schools ramped up, new black physicians increasingly graduated from predominantly white medical schools. Even after the opening of two additional black medical schools—Charles Drew (affiliated with UCLA) in 1966, and

Morehouse Medical School (in Atlanta) in 1978, black medical schools as a whole were only educating about 25 percent of all black medical students, and in the 1980s this figure dropped significantly.

Nonetheless, even with special programs at predominantly white medical schools running full throttle, growth in the supply of black physicians and other black healthcare professionals was exceedingly slow. The reality was that in 1970, for example, the 6,106 black physicians in the United States were just 2 percent of the total physicians and surgeons in a nation in which 11 percent of its population was black. As of 1980, the proportion of black physicians within the national physician supply was 3.1 percent. Ironically, at the same time, a widespread physician shortage beginning in the 1950s had led to an influx of foreign medical graduates filling employment gaps in the nation's hospitals.

During these decades of dramatic national integration of black healthcare professionals, black medical institutions like Meharry provided graduates who, in turn, bridged the medical establishment into black communities and patient populations. The work of Carl C. Bell, M.D., a prominent black psychiatrist in Chicago exemplifies the bridge-building black medical professional. A psychiatrist and public health specialist, Bell graduated from Meharry Medical College (1971) and trained in psychiatry at the Illinois State Psychiatric Institute in Chicago. Bell held positions at various health facilities in the mostly black South Side of Chicago. He also became a leading member of the medical community, including the head of the psychiatry section of the NMA. Bell's contributions to bridge-building medicine emerged early in his career in his work at Jackson Park Hospital and a large community mental health center, the Community Mental Health Council (CMHC). In his writings, he noted, in the 1970s "the South Side's mental health system infrastructure was extremely underdeveloped, and there were few alternatives to hospitalization in a state hospital." Shaping himself into a "community psychiatrist," Bell wrote that even at this early point in his career, "I felt it my mission to use our [hospital] resources—however limited—and develop a system to address the needs of the poor and underserved African-American population."[8]

Bell developed a plan by which emergency room psychiatric care could be administered to psychotic patients, thereby avoiding the need to admit them to hospital in-patient settings that might or might not be available. He fully developed this healthcare delivery model later in his many years as the head of the CMHC. The center became one of the nation's largest nonprofit community health centers. Bell also became a psychiatric expert on community violence, cultural sensitivity and racism, as well as the psychiatric misdiagnosis of the black mentally ill. Over recent decades, Bell has been an adviser on these issues on panels for the U.S. surgeon general and for Congress.

The decade between the late 1960s and late 1970s was the most energized period of black collective consciousness and militant politics since Reconstruction. In fact, historians like Manning Marable refer to it as the Second Reconstruction. The political fervor from the wider black freedom struggle spilled into the halls of the nation's medical institutions, as well. Two movements emerged largely from within the black and political activist communities themselves that had a huge impact on the urban healthcare system. One was the mass unionization drives of urban health workers. The second was the movement to establish safe women's healthcare and family planning services, especially for poor minority urban and rural communities. These movements drew upon local activist leadership, but also from some of the nation's most prominent black, white, multiethnic, and feminist civil rights leaders and progressives.

Like black medical professionals during the 1960s and 1970s, black allied healthcare workers experienced a pressure cooker of clashing old and new forms of racial discrimination. In the case of nonprofessional black health workers, racial conflicts and worker strikes frequently occurred. One of the pivotal figures in the equality movement launched by the growing numbers of black hospital workers was Coretta Scott King. She had been exposed to segregation and oppressive labor conditions as a child growing up in rural Alabama. Her mother had only a fourth grade education. Her father was a farm owner who at times suffered at the hands of local white ruffians. After attending Antioch College, Coretta became active in racial equality and justice causes both before and after her marriage to the Reverend Martin Luther King Jr. Mrs. King criticized U.S. foreign policies during the Kennedy and Johnson administrations. In 1961, she worked with the Women Strike for Peace, attending an international conference on nuclear disarmament in Geneva, Switzerland. In 1965, she participated in peace rallies, including a protest at the White House. After her husband's death in 1968, she became a vigorous leader in the national campaigns of the Southern Christian Leadership Conference (SCLC), speaking at the Poor People's Campaign during the summer of 1968.

In 1968, the New York City hospital workers' union, Local 1199, asked Coretta King to serve as the honorary chair of its national organizing committee. The 1199 union was established in the 1930s to organize drugstores. It had built ties with black workers' struggles as far back as 1936, when it was involved in a strike in Harlem drugstores. By the early 1960s, the union was organizing professional and technical health workers, and began organizing hospital workers to form its union base. The 1199 organization had always formed partnerships with the civil rights movement, using slogans such as "Freedom and Decent Jobs." Indeed, the union chartered a special train and sent one thousand of its members to participate in the 1963 March on Washington. Martin Luther King Jr. referred to 1199 as "my favorite union."[9]

Given their longtime link to civil rights causes, civil rights organizations joined in support of the union's campaigns. The National Urban League (NUL) and Congress of Racial Equality (CORE) first became involved in 1199 strikes and protests in the 1960s. So when, in the spring of 1969, Coretta Scott King, Rev. Ralph Abernathy, and other leaders of SCLC joined with 1199 to support striking hospital workers in Charleston, both the union and SCLC already had developed a history of partnerships within the broader civil rights movement.

During the winter of 1968, black LPNs and nurse's assistants experienced continuous harsh supervision, and some were even terminated. Several co-workers began to meet weekly to discuss their common work problems. After several months they decided to strike. The goal of the strike was to gain recognition for the newly organized union (Local 1199B), as well as higher wages and improved work conditions. On March 20, 1969, some 510 black health workers at the University of South Carolina's Medical College Hospi-

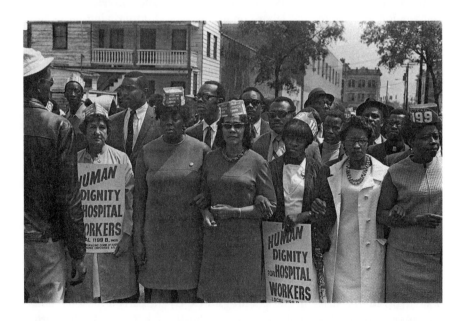

Figure 5.1.   Coretta Scott King leads a march in support of Charleston, South Carolina, hospital workers' strike, April 30, 1969. Mary Moultrie (left) and Rosetta Simmons (right), strike organizers, walk alongside Mrs. King. The strike lasted nearly three months.

Source: Adam Parker, "Local Hospital Workers' Courage Changed Workplaces Forever," *Charleston Post and Courier*, September 30, 2013. Photo by Dewey Swain.

tal (MCH) walked off the job. A week later, a group of 60 workers staged a similar walkout at a second public hospital, Charleston County Hospital. The overwhelming majority of the original striking workers (498 of 510) were women in lower-ranking, nonprofessional hospital occupations: LPNs, nurses' aides, and orderlies. SCLC considered the hospital worker union struggles as the second chapter of the Poor People's Campaign that they had conducted a year earlier.

In the Charleston strike, black women strikers and religious institutions became the backbone of the struggle. One energetic young worker in particular, Mary Moultrie, an LPN at the MCH, stood out. Moultrie spoke out for her coworkers who were most upset by the racial prejudice of their supervisors. White nursing and supervisory staff routinely belittled blacks employed as practical nurses and other service workers. Having returned to Charleston to work at MC Hospital following several years of hospital work in New York City, Moultrie discovered that even white nursing students would interact condescendingly with the black staff. Moultrie described her experience as common. Black nurses' aides would show the much younger white nursing students various aspects of nursing care. However, after "you'd teach them everything . . . if they wanted to say that you were a subordinate, they gave you an order and you didn't take it, [t]hey could fire you. You know, these are the 16, 17 and 18-year old nurse's students, but because they were white, they had that option." Gradually the nursing students exerted daily pressure on the black nurses' aides: "You know, you either did what they asked you to do, I mean told you to do or they could write you up, or they could even have you fired."[10]

Four weeks into the strike, SCLC committed its national leaders to travel to Charleston to support it. The most prominent of these leaders was Coretta Scott King, along with the Reverend Ralph Abernathy. At the time Coretta King was the nation's most popular civil rights figure, having endured the recent assassination of her husband under international media attention. Both Coretta King and Abernathy believed that the Charleston hospital strike was similar in moral significance to the Memphis sanitation workers strike. Each of these labor protests involved mostly black low-income strikers seeking redress for issues involving basic respect, as well as fair wages, benefits, and minimum job security for workers.

Coretta King headed a group of fourteen civil rights figures in support of the Charleston strike. This group included leaders of some of the nation's most influential civil rights organizations, as well as prominent political leaders such as New York's Representative Shirley Chisholm; president of the National Council of Negro Women, Dorothy Height; and executive director of the National Welfare Rights Organization, George A. Wiley. The group drew up a public statement urging the South Carolina governor to recognize the strikers' union: South Carolina's intransigence "tells much about what is wrong with America today." They called the Charleston strike "a fight for human rights and human dignity."[11]

Throughout the strike and protests, city police and state troopers patrolled the Charleston streets. At the request of the Charleston local police just a day or two before Reverend Abernathy's arrival in the city, the state of South Carolina also sent one thousand national guardsmen to monitor the strikers. The noted *New York Times* writer James Wooten reported the national guardsmen "lined up, two abreast, outside a church," wearing gas masks, with bayonets fixed, standing next to a small tank that was blocking street exits. One of the protesting youth described the situation as "a concentration camp, that is what it is."[12] The protesters were cornered into a two-block section. When the police ordered the protesters to disperse, and the protestors refused, the police arrested scores of them. Reverend Abernathy was among the 350 protesters arrested during the standoff, along with some 140 marching black youth and the two white priests who led the youth's march.[13]

In the meantime, Coretta Scott King became the public face for the Charleston strikers. Like Abernathy, she made a number of trips to the city to attend its rallies. Local black churches mobilized a large support base of community residents for the strikers. At one meeting, there were an estimated seven thousand Charleston residents in the audience, mostly black—about one-third of the city's overall black population.

The coalition between the 1199 organizers in Charleston and the local and national offices of SCLC injected a blend of Christian revivalism and union cries for economic justice into America's hospital establishment. In the spring of 1970, at the one-hundred-day mark of the strike, the *New York Times* reported: "[T]he experience of Local 1199 affords encouraging evidence that a racially integrated approach within existing institutions can redistribute power and thus begin to satisfy the yearnings of those in the cellar of opportunity for self-direction toward a place in the sun."[14]

The news of the struggle for racial justice by health workers in the hospitals of Charleston rippled out to other hospitals across the nation. The Charleston strike led to the formation of 1199 district chapters across the mid-Atlantic states, as well as in Kentucky and New Mexico. In 1974, and again in 1978, echoing the Charleston strike, the largely black service workers at the Duke University Medical Center conducted unionization drives.

To the poor black, Hispanic, and working-class white residents of cities, one of the most frustrating aspects of their healthcare situation was the abysmal lack of maternity health and family planning services. Illegal abortions were commonplace and took a high toll on women's lives in the urban poor areas. Furthermore, family planning services in city hospitals that serviced poor communities were often overcrowded and uninviting places. Many women in poor communities had strong reservations against using hospital family planning services. One mother of six in the Bronx (New York City) described the typical situation: "If you have ever been to the regular hospital clinics for family planning, where there are always crowds, and they never explain about the examinations and all, you would know why people are afraid of them."[15]

Around the country, there were highly publicized incidents in which poor black and Hispanic women had been sterilized, or lost their children as the result of harsh legal and welfare procedures. Furthermore, there were reports that some women in Puerto Rico were unknowingly sterilized. Consequently throughout inner-city black and Hispanic communities, fear and mistrust was widespread that hospitals were "butcher shops" in which women could experience unwanted sterilization.

Thus, black, Hispanic, and other poor women were caught in a dual dilemma. On the one hand, these women wanted family planning and maternity care resources. However, on the other hand, they were apprehensive about the motives, quality of care, and health effects they could expect at the hospitals and clinics in their communities. Upper-class black and white women could obtain safe abortions through private doctors, but poor women could not afford this treatment.

To address these issues, government health centers, urban hospitals, and academic hospitals with family planning and maternity care programs that served women in poor black and Hispanic neighborhoods enlisted community women themselves in the planning and provision of family healthcare services. These programs also employed black and Latina women as professional and nonprofessional staff. Most of the paraprofessionals and nurses' aides were from communities that the health centers served. These employees were effective in attracting community populations to use the center and to follow up on prenatal care and family planning measures. They also became part of the community of bridge-building black medical and health workers.

In order to establish successful family planning and prenatal services in urban poor areas, the OEO initiated programs in which hospitals and medical schools would link with neighborhood health center or services. Black and Hispanic women were included on planning groups that advised each center about reaching program objectives, as well as for screening staff for the program. In New York City, for example, family planning health programs were set up in a health center in the Bronx section of the city in partnership with Albert Einstein College of Medicine and the Bronx (Jacobi) Municipal Hospital Center. The program offered prenatal care, as well as examinations and free contraceptives.

Family health and planning programs were gradually reaching the inner-city poor. Nonetheless, battles against family planning clinics continued to occur from community to community, and from city to city. On one side were the traditional political and religious interests steadfastly opposed to family planning services of any sort. On the other hand, there were medical and social work professionals, feminists, and other women's groups bent on starting or expanding family planning resources in their communities. For example, in Louisiana, as late as 1964 it was a felony just to distribute information about family planning. In order for the state government to gain enough public support to start family planning services, it conducted extensive surveys that corroborated the need for and women's interest in family planning. The surveys revealed an estimated 130,000 medically indigent women were in need of family planning resources. By 1969, family planning services were available in only thirty-three of the state's sixty-four parishes (or counties).

In New York City a distinctive family planning program centered on using peer women in the counseling process. The incorporation of nonprofessional women from the hospital community to enhance enrollment and follow-up of community women made this program distinct. By 1970, fifty-one such counselors were employed by twenty-three hospitals throughout the city. Each counselor met with from five to ten women per day, and they had interviewed an estimated 2,800 patients per month.

The expansion of family planning services into poor urban communities in the late 1960s ran into public and political opposition. Family planning initiatives often set aflame an intense conflict between women health advocates and the medical establishment. There was growing concern over the frequent destructive effects of poorly tested contraceptive devices and procedures. As pediatrician and public health activist Helen Rodriguez-Trias has written, "[a]s the reports of deadly complications of pills and IUDs grew, so did women's anger at being used."[16] The situation in the black community was no less tense. In Louisiana officials had to combat "a counter-force" widespread among the poor, especially the black poor. These segments were suspicious of government family planning projects, believing these programs were "concealing a hidden agenda to coerce the poor through such measures as punitive sterilization, deprivation of welfare, seizure of children, and even jailing of unwed parents."[17] Black nationalists were especially critical of family planning services that targeted poorer black women. Radical organizations such as the Black Panthers and the Young Lords pointed to the experimental contraception programs that had been imposed on their racial and ethnic groups, calling them a form of racial genocide.

Despite divisions within black communities across the country, family planning resources increased during the 1970s. Black women in particular took the lead on this issue, as healthcare professionals and policymakers, as organizers, and as activists. Each year reproductive healthcare became increasingly central in the new healthcare network shaped by the federal government.

Popular black militancy and strong progressive political leaders and journalism also made the 1970s the ripe time for a public attack on the federal government's Tuskegee Syphilis Study (TSS). The Congressional Black Caucus (CBC) was among the most vociferous critics of the study. Founded in 1971, and comprised of thirteen black members of Congress, the CBC gradually grew into a force supporting the health equality drives emanating from the black communities nationwide, among other issues. The new presence of the CBC in Washington, DC, gave blacks a seat at the federal legislative table. There the group was poised to expose any egregious instances and practices of medical racism, as well as to plan and advocate specific governmental remedies.

On July 26, 1972, just a year after the CBC was formed, the *New York Times* dropped a medical bombshell with its front-page headline: "Syphilis Victims in U.S. Study Went Untreated for 40 years," by reporter Jean Heller. Other disclosures rippled throughout the nation's black and white press and television news. *Ebony* magazine, America's most widely circulating black American popular magazine, carried an article on the TSS titled "Condemned to Die for Science." Within days of the initial news report about TSS, the CBC and the NAACP placed strong pressure on the federal government to halt the study. Consequently, the Department of Health, Education, and Welfare (HEW) formed the Tuskegee Syphilis Study Ad Hoc Advisory Panel. Among its members were prominent black Americans from the professional and medical communities, who were in concert with the militant activism pervading black communities at this time. The Committee also included an interracial cluster of advocates in law, medical ethics, and public service with expertise in protecting the rights of patients and other disadvantaged groups such as the mentally ill and disabled. The chair of the panel was Dr. Broadus N. Butler, the head of the National Negro College Fund. Other key members included the prominent theologian Seward Hiltner, and Attorney Ronald H. Brown, the general counsel for the National Urban League, who later served as the campaign manager for Senator Edward Kennedy and Reverend Jesse Jackson.

In April 1973, the Final Report of the TSS Ad Hoc Advisory Panel was transmitted to HEW. The report summarized the utter condemnation the group leveled at the government-medical researchers: "There is ample evidence in the records [we reviewed] that the consent to participation was not obtained from the Tuskegee Syphilis Study subjects, but that instead they were exploited, manipulated, and deceived. They were treated not as human subjects but as objects of research."[18]

Not surprisingly the Panel recommended the TSS "be terminated immediately" and that "the participants involved in the study . . . [b]e given the care now required to treat any disabilities resulting from their participation."[19] The public anger concerning TSS was so strong that Congress began hearings to investigate the abuse of patients and medical care more broadly. The result of these hearings was the passage of the National Medical Research Act of 1974, which shaped federal policies protecting patients from unethical medical experimentation. An official apology was made some two decades later (see photo).

Aside from attacking the TSS, black community activists also helped to bring national attention to black sickle cell disease sufferers as a health equality issue. In 1970, the federal government estimated that between twenty-five thousand and fifty thousand black Americans had the disease. Life for thousands of them meant living with various disabilities and intense pain. In addition, some two million blacks had the sickle cell trait, and as many as one thousand black infants were born with the disease each year. In the late 1960s and early 1970s, there was growing public dissatisfaction with the neglect of black America's sickle cell disease problem. Medical and public health professionals and workers with black patient populations affected by sickle cell disease were particularly agitated about this negligence. The Congressional Black Caucus, civil rights organizations, and other activists criticized government authorities publicly for their lack of concern for this health

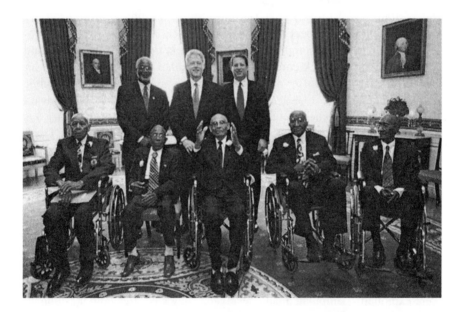

Figure 5.2.   White House apology ceremony for the participants and survivors of the Tuskegee Syphilis Study, May 16, 1997. Surgeon General David Satcher is standing beside President Bill Clinton and Vice President Al Gore.

Source: White House Photography Office 1997, accessed August 31, 2017, at http:// tuskegeestudy.weebly.com/clintons-apology.html.

issue, as did groups like the Black Panthers who were conducting grassroots sickle cell programs in black communities. Civil rights activist and member of the Georgia House of Representatives Julian Bond led the effort to pass a state law covering sickle cell, requiring the state and county public health departments to provide sickle cell testing programs. By 1972, twelve states required testing of infants for sickle cell. Although many blacks still feared that an emphasis on sickle cell disease could make blacks targets of discrimination based on genetic racism, these measures indicated the growing public interest in reducing sickle cell anemia.

Finally, President Nixon and other federal leaders responded to the pressure with the passage of the National Sickle Cell Anemia Control Act of 1972. Since taking office in 1969, Nixon believed strongly that the nation's health system was in need of a fundamental rebuilding. In 1971, his National Health Strategy proposal to Congress included $6 million in funds for sickle cell research and treatment. When Nixon signed the Sickle Cell Act into law on May 16, 1972, he hoped to assure the public, "[t]hese actions make clear, I believe, the urgency with which this country is working to alleviate and arrest the suffering from this disease."[20]

During the 1960s and 1970s, the federal government was pushed to the lead in bringing millions of blacks into the nation's medical care system, as well as improving living conditions for the black and minority poor. By the mid-1970s, black health leaders had achieved many of their major goals. Medicaid and Medicare, along with federally aided hospitals and community health centers, greatly improved access to medical care for black Americans, along with other largely poor and elderly populations. Between 1964 and 1976, physician visits for poor children almost doubled, and for poor adults and poor elderly, it increased by 33 and 18 percent respectively. Black medical leaders had helped to develop greater access for blacks to medical institutions, neighborhood health centers, and family and women's health services. They also expanded hospital unions to better the working conditions for black hospital workers. In short, during the 1960s and 1970s, the movement for black health equality had spread into many corners of the nation's medical landscape. But the question remained: Was this successful surge toward health equality for and by blacks sustainable in the last quarter of the twentieth century?

Many of the Battlers who had emerged among black medical professionals during the civil rights era took on bridge-building roles for the nation's medical establishment during the 1970s and early 1980s. While these black health professionals worked as conciliatory links between predominantly white healthcare institutions and black communities and patient populations, a core of New Activists would emerge in the later 1980s to further challenge these institutions. Their interests lay more in exposing racial healthcare disparities, as well as injustices in social and political conditions that negatively affected local and national black community health. They were concerned with using medical institutions, health agencies, and health programs to address the deep-rooted social inequities and injustices they believed underlay black America's medical and public health problems.

Chapter Six

Confronting the Black Health Crisis

By the mid-1970s, the health equality ideal had reached a high point of national interest. Unlike the post–Civil War Freedmen's Bureau, the New Deal initiatives, or the Hill-Burton program, this time the presidents, Congress, and major federal agencies *believed in* and committed nationwide resources to improve the health of blacks and other American minorities. They also expanded opportunities in all parts of the country for blacks to enter medical care institutions as professionals and allied health personnel, as well as community health leaders and advisers.

In the late 1960s and early 1970s, millions of the poor—especially blacks, other racial minorities, the elderly, and disabled Americans—had benefited from the War on Poverty as well as federal civil rights and health insurance programs. Also, affirmative action policies mandated by federal and state governments had begun to turn the tide in the integration of blacks into medical schools, hospitals, and health agencies. The number of blacks in the nation's medical education pipeline and hospital employment fields expanded substantially. Indeed, as in public education and voting, a Second Reconstruction had occurred in the federal support for healthcare. Medicare and Medicaid made admission of the disadvantaged to hospitals for initial treatment a national practice by the 1970s. Blacks were admitted as new patients to hospitals of all types and sizes across the nation. Throughout America's massive healthcare sector, the liberal nation-state goal of racial integration had moved apace with integration of the nation's other major institutions.

However, starting in the mid-1970s, a nationwide "black health crisis" began to unfold. At this time, major health agencies and medical research bodies noted continuing black-white health disparities in their surveys. For example, between 1965 and 1975, death rates for blacks compared to whites for major chronic diseases such as heart disease and hypertension were three and seven times higher for blacks, respectively. This black health crisis became even more evident during the Ronald Reagan presidency. The nation's urban landscape was changing, as concentrated poverty or "New Ghettos" took shape. In these inner-city areas, struggles to eliminate the critical health and medical care problems of black and Hispanic residents compared to their white urban and suburban counterparts became an arduous seemingly endless affair. Moreover, nationwide black Americans had to deal with two new major epidemics—AIDS and rampant drug addiction—spreading throughout their communities.

During the 1980s and 1990s, New Activists emerged from the black healthcare and political communities to take on the black health crisis. In order to cut away at black health disparities and community health problems, New Activists replaced the goals of the Battlers. They shifted beyond the integrationist legal and policy struggles of the bygone civil rights era. New Activists also went beyond just the role of bridge-building to improve black patient care and community input occurring at predominantly white-run institutions. Instead, they struggled to shape resources from within black communities themselves, and not just from the nation's larger medical establishment. The new black community self-help focus came about to address the morally charged aspects of the AIDS crisis. It also was necessary because the healthcare system did little to support black communities facing environmental racism and intransigent poverty. Indeed, the New Activists were destined to struggle against three large-scale public health menaces in particular: medical needs produced by urban poverty and pollution, the AIDS epidemic, and medical care gaps, even collapses, due to natural disasters.

In 1976, at the Atlanta University–hosted national W. E. B. Du Bois Conference on black health, Dr. J. Alfred Cannon, head of psychiatry at the Charles R. Drew School of Medicine, warned of the coming crisis in black America. A political backlash against the policies and programs that had led to so much black health progress and collective well-being had begun. "Black America is in deep economic, psychological, social and spiritual distress," he told attendees. "The 'highs' of the 1960s, when blacks were at the epicenter of this nation's conscience and led the humanitarian revolution, are over. . . . Blacks who had national and international visibility, relevance and significance, are now on the backwaters of progress." The social progress blacks had experienced in the previous decade had not been sufficient to eliminate the historic burdens that blacks bore. "Events prior to and following the 1960s have caused severe trauma to the black community," he explained, "and the depth of the violation is such as to now pose, more seriously than before, the question of *the very survival of black America.*"[1]

By the 1980s, changing patterns of poverty and political conflict in large urban and rural black communities were emerging along with a "black health crisis." The term was shorthand for the excessive levels of mortality and public health problems afflicting blacks. It also referred to the growing wave of closings of community hospitals and socioeconomic barriers preventing vulnerable groups within the black community from access to adequate healthcare. In city after city, statistics revealed steady or growing health disparities between blacks and other racial minorities, on the one hand, and whites, on the other. For black Americans, the health problems of the black poor families and their children were the most intense and intransigent. These problems were directly linked to a poor standard of living, joblessness, incarceration, and homelessness. Blacks in the lower and middle classes faced the problem of disorganized care and insufficient preventive medicine. Blacks as a whole, like the nation's other disadvantaged minority populations, lacked ample screening and appropriate treatment for a variety of medical problems, such as cancers, heart diseases, STDs, and mental illness. Furthermore, the quality of care for blacks, especially mothers and children, despite government health insurance for the poorest segments, tended to be significantly lower than for whites of similar economic and educational status.

Health activists traced the deficiencies in black health status and medical care resources directly to government cutbacks in social welfare and public health programs and funding. Most damaging were the reductions in funds for urban public hospitals that served high concentrations of the black poor, minority poor, and disabled populations. Also, in the South, some state legislatures worked diligently to freeze or limit the inflow of federal health dollars that would open greater access to medical services for their poor black populations. Conservative legislators and governors in the South used a variety of ways to block as much federal Medicaid funding as possible. This relieved these states from providing their share of funds for the medical services received by the Medicaid recipients.

In its early phase, the federal government established a simple requirement for Medicaid eligibility: An applicant merely needed to certify that he or she was a recipient of public welfare. However, in the South the income criteria for public welfare eligibility was set so low that hundreds of thousands of poor people throughout the South, who, by federal standards, were below the poverty line, were still ineligible for Medicaid. In some Southern states, Medicaid and Medicare funds paid for private, for-profit hospital beds and nursing homes at the expense of building community and outpatient primary care resources needed by local underserved populations. Public community and ambulatory services would have been more effective for improving the health of poorer communities.

As public health historian E. Richard Brown observed, Medicaid and Medicare so to speak "awakened the Leviathan," fueling a constant rise in medical costs. The "injection of public monies into the largely private medical market provided what seemed like unlimited revenues for physicians and private hospitals."[2] Medical providers set up policies and practices, raising prices as necessary, that favored the wealthier, privately insured patient population. At the same time, poorer blacks, people of color, and women were marginalized to rudimentary care or even not treated at all. As of the mid-1970s, only 6 percent of the nation's doctors were treating one-third of the Medicaid patients; some physicians were employed at hospitals that discouraged Medicaid patient care; and one-fifth of doctors nationwide did not see Medicaid patients at all.

In 1983, Harold Washington, Chicago's first African American mayor, addressed the NMA at its national convention. He zeroed in on the inadequate hospital resources for the urban needy, a condition he argued was compounded by the flaws in the Medicaid and Medicare system. Washington, one of the nation's most prominent black elected politicians, lamented that these public health insurance funds were being used directly for growing private hospital chains and other for-profit medical services. In the meantime, he pointed out, "As health costs run wild, the poor, many of them black, are being shrugged out of private hospitals" only to be "dumped in greater numbers each year on the struggling public hospitals, such as Cook County Hospital here in Chicago."[3]

The deficiencies in inner-city medical resources that fueled the black health crisis were coupled with the emergence of the New Ghetto—namely impoverished social and neighborhood conditions. The weakening of tens of thousands of urban black families, their unhealthy physical environment, and the decline of jobs inside black communities were all key cornerstones of the New Ghetto and the black health crisis landscape. The health crisis and the New Ghetto were inextricably linked—the twin protagonists in the troubling chapter in modern black health and medical care history.

In the latter 1970s and early 1980s, large clusters of neighborhoods began showing signs of environmental decline. Aggravating the spread of poverty was a process that urban social scientists and geographers call "desertification." With the speed-up of suburbanization and disappearance of employment spreading throughout the nation's major cities, desertification was the wide-scale abandonment of large tracts of housing and industrial sites in cities. Blocks of residential housing were emptying out as mostly white working-class and middle-income families moved to the suburbs. Jobs also were flooding away from the cities as corporations relocated their management and factories to suburban locations or to far-off regions or even to foreign countries. As the revenue base in the black and Latino inner-city sections left behind declined, so did city public services. Poverty intensified. Municipal services such as police, sanitation, and firefighting declined. Burned-out buildings and poorly lit streets attracted transient populations desperate for accessible places to congregate and live. Desertification also was causally linked to increasing levels of violent crime and drug abuse in neighborhoods.

Beginning in the late 1980s, the growing black middle class also started to physically break off from the traditional black community neighborhoods, and an estimated seven million moved to the suburbs between 1970 and 1995. Most moved to predominantly white neighborhoods. However, a substantial population moved into racially separated black enclaves in the suburbs. Although largely middle class, many among these enclaves maintained mobile ties with family, churches, and social networks still located in traditional inner-city communities. Another substantial portion of the new black middle class of the 1980s remained living in close proximity to housing and public projects inhabited by the low-income black poor. In fact, during the 1980s and 1990s, overall residential segregation in most U.S. cities remained the same or intensified.

By the early 1980s, nearly 60 percent of blacks lived in central cities. These urban neighborhoods had the nation's highest rates of many preventable diseases, young and young adult deaths due to violence, and populations lacking adequate housing and/or health insurance. Indeed, in the 1980s and 1990s, public policymakers and national media referred to the residents of these impoverished black and minority neighborhoods as the nation's "underclass."

In these conditions, mass erosion of traditional black urban families and neighborhood life started to appear. Between 1960 and 1970, the proportion of black families with children born to unmarried women increased from 22 percent to 35 percent, compared to 3 and 6 percent for white families. By 1980, this proportion rose to 55 percent compared to 11 percent for whites. Teenage pregnancy rates for black girls were twice the rates of whites. Leading sociologists Joyce Ladner and Ruby Gourdine noted that the wave of adolescent pregnancies sweeping America was black and white. However, "[f]or African-Americans, the problem of teenage pregnancy is particularly devastating because of the [serious] sociomedical consequences experienced by this group."[4] The biggest challenge for family members in these single-parent families was poverty. As one Southern health expert wrote, the single-mother families "lived lives of such impoverishment and physical and social isolation that they were largely invisible to those health agencies, doctors, and political leaders who had the means to help them."[5] By 1985, about two-thirds of the children living in black households headed by single women were in poverty.

Concentrated poverty in major urban and rural black communities made maintaining healthcare programs in these areas difficult. Often households either lacked educated, health-conscious parents or sufficient funds for and physical proximity to low-cost primary care and nutritional guidance. Physical environments including unsafe housing, traffic pollution, and psychological stressors such as neighborhood violence added to the residents' physical and psychological health burdens.

Nationally, beginning in the mid-1970s, more than two times as many black mothers had no or little prenatal care compared to white mothers, and twice as many black babies as white were low birth weight at birth. Low birth weight for babies is associated with high infant mortality and also indicates inadequate prenatal care resources. In 1986, 18 of every 1,000 black babies died within the first year of life, and nearly 13 percent suffered from low birth weight. As Byllye Avery, the founding president of the National Black Women's Health Project stated, these "infant mortality data suggest that African Americans constitute an almost entirely separate class of people in this country, and that this de facto segregation is a violation of basic human and civil rights."[6]

The black health crisis of the late 1970s and 1980s was a major factor in the shift by black voters from pursuing traditional civil rights goals and protests to seeking gains in local electoral politics. Black voters reasoned that to improve policy in health, education, courts, and human services, they themselves had to have influence within the decision-making leaders and managers of city institutions, including hospitals and health agencies. Reaching a high point in the 1980s and 1990s, voters in cities with significant black populations concentrated on winning elections of black mayors. In city after city, furious campaign battles pitted a local black candidate popular in the black and liberal communities against a conventional white candidate usually drawn from the city political machine. Black mayoral candidates won in scores of small and large cities throughout the nation, including Cleveland, Atlanta, Chicago, Los Angeles, and New York City.

In step with the heightened political involvement of blacks in cities, many New Activist health leaders made training medical personnel to meet the black health crisis head-on a high priority. In Los Angeles, area authorities started the Charles Drew School of Medicine (affiliated with UCLA) in the aftermath of the Watts Riots of 1965, as well as Martin Luther King Jr. General Hospital (built in 1972) especially for underserved populations of the city. Morehouse Medical School (in Atlanta) opened in 1978. In the early 1980s, the number of both hospital-based and community-based medical services Drew Medical School provided skyrocketed. By 1984, the institution treated some 60,000 trauma cases annually and oversaw 6,000 births. While they treated people of all ethnicities, most of these patients were black and Hispanic. In addition, the medical school operated over twenty community programs. Many, such as Head Start, focused on pediatric services and healthy child development.[7]

While schools like Drew and Morehouse were performing valiantly to reduce the serious black health differentials surfacing in inner cities throughout the nation, the structure of medical education as a whole was being pulled toward a "colorblind" model of selecting, training, and placing medical professionals. Black medical schools still educated about 25 percent of all black medical students as of 1982. But nationally, since the mid-1960s, in response to the nation's racial discord, predominantly white medical and dental schools had embarked on affirmative action programs, and the percent of black medical students attending these schools had been steadily increasing. Surveys revealed black physicians provided the most physician care to the nation's black communities and patient populations. Consequently, medical schools like the University of California attempted to contribute their share of newly educated black physicians. The University of California-Davis opened a new medical school in 1966 to meet growing healthcare needs and started an affirmative action program to attract black and Latino students. By the year 2000, only about 15 percent of black medical students were in the black schools, with this percentage declining still in the early years of the twenty-first century.

However, the pipelines that generated black health personnel met with political obstacles. Even as the black health crisis and New Ghetto poverty spread, political conservatism threatened to reduce the supply of black health professionals. National political backlash surfaced in opposition to affirmative action initiatives in the medical sector. This backlash came to a head with the U.S. Supreme Court case *Regents of the University of California v. Bakke*.

Allan P. Bakke was a white male candidate for admission to the University of California at Davis Medical School. When the school denied him admission twice, despite a superior academic record and Medical College Admissions Test (MCAT) scores, he sued the University in the California court system. His suit charged that the University employed a dual-track admissions program—one for blacks and other racial minorities, the other for the white majority—that violated the U.S. and California constitutions, as well as Title VI of the Civil Rights Act. In 1978, the U.S. Supreme Court ruled that the special admissions program for blacks and other minorities was unconstitutional and unfair to Mr. Bakke. In two separate five-to-four majority opinions, the court ordered that UC-Davis admit Bakke to its medical school. This majority opinion found that the program violated the equal protection clause of the Fourteenth Amendment. While the Court barred racial quotas and the use of race as a primary factor for future admission to the school, in the second majority opinion, it ruled race-conscious remedies in admissions procedures were constitutional in situations in which the government had established specific past discrimination, which was not the case at the newly created UC-Davis Medical School.

The *Bakke* ruling reduced the number of blacks admitted throughout the nation's medical schools. In a small number of "top tier" medical schools, the admission of black students remained a significant priority. However, in the nation's middle- and lower-ranked schools, the percentage of blacks admitted dropped to or remained at miniscule levels. *Bakke*, along with similar Supreme Court cases in this period, diverted the nation's medical establishment from attempting structural changes to medical education and professionalization. Policies and programs like that at the University of California at Davis were designed in part to improve the supply of black and minority doctors, nurses, and other health professionals for medically needy urban and rural communities. Now, as the nation came under the leadership of the Reagan administration, many conservatives viewed special minority programs as racially patronizing—that is, "reverse racism" against white Americans.

Despite the *Bakke* controversy, many affirmative action initiatives continued into the 1980s. Beneficiaries of special minority programs, many black health professionals and technicians joined the health fields alongside other minorities. These included talented upper-class black Americans, as well as international students and medical personnel immigrating to the United States. Many from these streams of minority healthcare personnel—black descendants of American slavery and foreign backgrounds—moved into the front lines of hospitals and health agencies that cared for the nation's growing urban black and minority poor populations. Depending on the city and state, large if not dominant portions of their patients were recipients of Medicaid and Medicare as the sole or major source of health insurance. As such, these healthcare institutions were essential to providing basic aspects of care to minority communities.

In 1970, the American Association of Medical Colleges had set a goal for minority medical school enrollment of 12 percent of the nation's total enrollment by 1980. However, as of 1987, just 3 percent of the nation's physicians were black, and 6 percent of medical students; this despite the fact that blacks still comprised 12 percent of the nation's population. For black American medical providers, there was also growing competition from increasing numbers of foreign-nationality physicians, especially from African and Caribbean nations. In 1990, foreign-born physicians comprised nearly one-fourth of the nation's black female physicians, and one-fifth of the nation's doctors overall. The global flow of foreign-background nursing talent into the U.S. medical workforce accelerated, as well. Together, foreign-source and black American nurses formed a bulk of the personnel who worked inside the medical care network for poor urban black communities.

Along with global trends, increased opportunities for women were reshaping the black and minority physician sectors throughout the nation. Around this time labor experts noted that a "gender revolution" was occurring in the nation's physician workforce. Between 1980 and 1990, the physician workforce grew from 431,000 to 586,000, a nearly 38 percent increase. The percentage of women physicians expanded from 13.3 percent in 1980 to

20 percent in 1990. The increase in the number of black women physicians was even more pronounced. In 1980, they amounted to 25 percent of the black physicians. This rose to over 33 percent in 1990. Moreover, black women made up about 44 percent of the black physicians under the age of thirty-four in 1990.

The new black physicians of the late 1980s and 1990s clustered mainly in the primary care specialties—that is, family or general practice, pediatrics, or general internal medicine. Moreover black physicians tended to serve primarily black and poor patients. On average for younger black physicians, more than half of their patients were black, a rate five times higher than that of other young physicians. Furthermore, blacks specialized in obstetrics/gynecology at twice the rates of other minorities and whites, an important factor in addressing maternal health issues. These new generations of black physicians and other health professionals were scattered racially and functionally throughout the complex organizational structures of hospitals and clinics. This was unlike the preintegration generations of old, in which blacks in medicine tended to work together in black health institutions and community settings.

By the mid-1980s, national spending within the medical care sector had grown so large that it rivaled the nation's education and defense budgets. The bulk of the nation's hospitals were operated by government, large private companies, nonprofit bodies, and not-for-profit healthcare businesses such as Kaiser Permanente. In this context, the Black Medical World as a healthcare network for black geographical communities had long faded away. Frozen out of government, corporate, and nonprofit economic circles, most black hospitals in cities were shuttered, merged into larger hospital systems, or renovated into facilities like nursing homes. In 1979, Homer G. Phillips Hospital in St. Louis, formerly one of the nation's largest producers of black physicians and nurses, closed. In 1987, Chicago's famous Provident Hospital and Nurses Training School, which for nearly a century had been a mainstay in the Black Medical World, also closed its doors.

The Achievers and Battlers earlier in the twentieth century had strong links to black health facilities, black medical and nursing schools, and black commercial districts and neighborhoods. By contrast, most black health professionals of the 1980s and 1990s were employed within the mainstream medical care establishment. This establishment blanketed cities, suburbs, and rural counties. It was comprised of a vast, essentially unorganized spread of hundreds of spatially disconnected medical facilities. Nonetheless, from among the ranks of the black medical professionals in the cities with substantial black populations, New Activists emerged. These black health professionals and lay health workers maintained a strong sense of collective identity and community commitment. Along with their foreign-background, new American counterparts, New Activists could be found as clinical staff managers and allied health personnel throughout the "safety net" healthcare sector.

The safety net resource was the informal network of public hospitals, emergency room services, and community health facilities located in or near poor minority neighborhoods in the large cities and towns. Other safety net facilities included neighborhood health services run by city and state health departments; small-group physician practices; and family planning services. Finally, the safety net resources included community-based free or sliding-scale clinics and outreach programs. These programs were designed to serve specific groups unreachable by hospital programs who were especially vulnerable to health problems such as domestic abuse or neighborhood violence. Many of these small programs were operated in small buildings or as mobile units by nonprofit and grassroots activist organizations.

As the storms of the black health crisis, poverty, and black political stridency in America's major cities grew, some federal health authorities evaluated more thoroughly the health and healthcare issues of black Americans nationwide. In 1983, Margaret M. Heckler, the secretary of the Department of Health and Human Services (DHHS), reacted to the glaring statistical pattern running through surveys of the health of Americans: the historical chasm between the health of blacks, Hispanics, Asian/Pacific Islanders, and Native Americans compared to that of whites. She called racial differences in health "an affront both to our ideals and to the ongoing genius of American medicine."[8]

To take stock of the DHHS's current data and activities relating to minority health and illuminate root causes for the minority-white health disparities, Heckler created the Secretary's Task Force on Black and Minority Health, composed of health specialists within federal agencies with expertise on black and minority health problems. This core subcommittee solicited presentations and survey information from hundreds of nonfederal organizations and individuals with particular knowledge about health issues of blacks and the other racial minority groups.

The Heckler task force found that death rates for blacks exceeded those of whites in six disease or health problem categories: accidents and homicides; infant mortality; heart disease and stroke; cirrhosis; cancer; and diabetes. The report, issued in 1985, woke up many of the nation's health policymakers as well as medical leaders to black and minority medical needs. It recommended changes in several areas of federal agency activities and the programs DHHS operated. These included improving the use of health information, education, and data; development of health professionals for needy minority groups; and a new research agenda relating to disparities. In addition, as a follow-up to the report, in 1987 DHHS established the Office of Minority Health (OMH), which was reauthorized by the Affordable Care Act in 2010. The OMH provides policy support, program development, and lead-

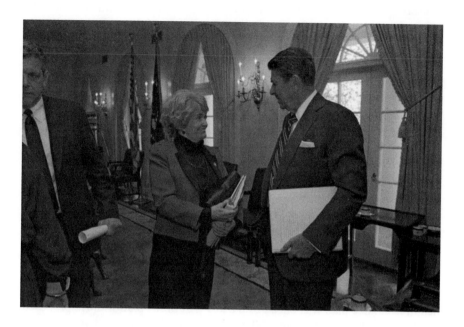

Figure 6.1.   Margaret M. Heckler, Secretary of Health and Human Services, with President Ronald W. Reagan, 1985.

Source: Courtesy of the Ronald Reagan Presidential Library.

ership training to healthcare agencies and communities. It advises DHHS and other federal agencies on issues related to minority health. These measures were designed in particular to close gaps in the health status of blacks and other minorities.

The Heckler Report served as a seminal guidebook for federal agencies addressing black and minority health disparities. It alerted personnel at these health agencies, as well as the hospitals and medical specialists serving minority patients and public health workers, about the root causes beneath the distinct health problems of the nation's blacks and other minorities. However, the report alone could not motivate the nation's healthcare delivery institutions to address the myriad black and minority group medical needs. Like the past struggles to integrate medical schools and hospitals, the challenge to close the health gaps unearthed by the Heckler Report fell heavily on the civil rights and political sectors.

With some thirty-five million Americans lacking health insurance in the early 1980s, black and white progressive political leaders once again took up the quest to pressure the federal government to establish universal healthcare coverage. This political movement attracted the New Activists of the black healthcare sector. It brought together populist Democrats, worker organizations, religious and social work organizations, as well as health activists into a forceful national constituency led by the Reverend Jesse Jackson. In his 1984 bid for the Democratic Party presidential nomination, Jackson included a national health insurance plan in his campaign platform. However, upon his defeat, the plan was removed from the Democratic Party's national platform.

In the following three years, the Reagan administration reduced federal health expenditures substantially. By 1986, about 36 percent of American children had no form of health insurance. Some analysts also estimated that over one-half of blacks living at poverty- or below poverty-level and about two-thirds of Hispanics of similar low-income groups lacked health insurance during all or part of the year. The availability and quality of medical care services delivered also had many deficiencies. For example, in 1986 approximately one-third of the nation's black women and one-fifth of white women did not receive adequate prenatal care. At the same time, costs for healthcare were also accelerating markedly. As of 1987, national costs for medical care amounted to 11.2 percent of the nation's gross national product, and were estimated to be growing 8.9 percent each year.

When Jesse Jackson reignited his presidential run in 1988, a national health insurance plan was once again a key part of his platform. He proposed the National Health Program (NHP), a policy of comprehensive, government-based healthcare insurance. It would replace "our wasteful, public-private patchwork medical delivery system," he said in a public speech while campaigning.[9] The program called for the eventual elimination of the current government, corporate, and health insurance bureaucracies. Under Reverend Jackson's health program, NHP benefits would replace the plans operated by some 1,500 private health insurance companies. The president and Congress would convene a national health board to administer the NHP. All citizens and residents of the United States would receive NHP insurance coverage, and the NHP would directly pay hospitals and health centers an annual budget based on the population and healthcare needs each facility served.

NHP insurance would cover the entire range of a person's medical care needs. This would include acute, emergency, and chronic care; home care; mental health and dental care; prescription drugs; and medical supplies. The NHP would also provide resources for preventive and public health services for communities. Funds for the NHP would derive from several sources. First, since the NHP would administer payments to healthcare providers, the administrative costs both of current public and private plans, as well as within hospitals, would be greatly reduced. In addition, company and individual payments to private insurance companies would go to the NHP, as well. Finally, the NHP program would obtain additional revenue from an increase in personal taxes on those with incomes in the upper-middle-class or wealthy ranges.

Public agitation for the single-payer health insurance system that Reverend Jackson championed all but disappeared from the national political scene when Jackson again lost the race for Democratic presidential nominee. The federal government proceeded with a mixed public-private health insurance policy known as managed care, which allowed private health insurance and providers to form health maintenance organizations (HMOs). These medical practices coordinated both the finance and delivery of healthcare with the intention of controlling costs while at the same time providing quality care to HMO enrollees. In this new period of market-oriented health insurance, the quest for healthcare equality fell to the NMA and individual politicians, especially those within the Congressional Black Caucus. With most of its membership experiencing aspects of the black health crisis on a daily basis, the NMA put its focus on bringing more healthcare resources into black communities no matter how financing was organized.

By the late 1980s, the political stirrings of black mayoral races as well as the impact of Jesse Jackson's Rainbow Coalition movement were fading. Elected officials, black health and community leaders, and religious-based activists in major cities were confronting the black health crisis along with a sea of other social and economic problems. They relied on the largely disorganized "safety net" healthcare sector to meet the medical needs produced by the black health crisis and other gaps in the citywide healthcare system. Municipalities also provided extra funding to safety net institutions so that these facilities could remain financially viable.

In the meantime, blocks of residential housing were emptying out of working-class and middle-income families. This population, mostly white but also black and Latino, was moving to the suburbs. Jobs also were flowing from the cities as corporations relocated their management and factories to suburban locations or other regions, or even to foreign countries. As the revenue base for cities declined, so did city public services. Yet at the same time, two major new health problems, the AIDS crisis and the crack cocaine epidemic, were starting to overwhelm the already overstressed municipal health systems.

In the early 1980s, physicians in Los Angeles, San Francisco, and New York began encountering cases of rare lung infections and severe immune deficiency among small numbers of previously healthy men. These cases were reported to the CDC. By the mid-1980s, the agency and other epidemiology centers established that a serious outbreak of AIDS was occurring nationwide and in other parts of the world, especially Africa.

In these early years of the AIDS outbreak, the nature and scope of this potential epidemic was still largely unclear to medical and public health authorities both nationally and across the globe. AIDS in the United States was referred to in popular stereotypical parlance as the "gay men's disease." The historic prejudice against gays and widespread homophobia resulted in many in the nation viewing gay Americans as an "invisible minority." The public mistakenly singled out this gay minority, saying they had brought the disease on themselves through their actions. Likely as a result, government health agencies like the CDC and FDA, reinforced by the Reagan administration's refusal to even publicly mention the disease until 1985, responded lethargically in seeking clinical treatments and urgent medical facilities for gay patients.

As the decade wore on, AIDS began to strike blacks and other racial minorities heavily, especially their gay and so-called IV (for intravenous) drug user subpopulations. Still, health policymakers essentially downplayed the severity of the disease's effects on the gays and other minority group segments. Throughout much of the 1980s, it was left up to the local gay and grassroots charitable organizations, as well as the gay underground alternative health caretakers, to provide a network of homes and living-assistance workers. The gay communities throughout the nation also developed alternative treatments based on their collective networks and experiences with AIDS. These treatments were used for those who had the HIV virus but were not experiencing symptoms or to care for those already sickened by AIDS.

In the meantime, the AIDS picture in black communities also was rapidly changing from bad to worse. AIDS deaths among black males increased on average 300 per 100,000 population each year during the late 1980s. Year by year, the proportion of blacks among the nation's AIDS victims rose steadily. In 1984, there were about 7,000 AIDS cases in the United States. Whites comprised 59 percent of these cases, blacks 25 percent, and Hispanics 14 percent. The annual death for black males rose to three times that of white males by 1988. Within the next seven years, for the first time in the epidemic's history, both the number and percentage of blacks with AIDS exceeded those of whites. Blacks made up 41 percent of all AIDS cases compared to 38 percent for whites.

The second epidemic to strike the nation's poorer communities and minorities of color came from a rise in the illegal drug trade. During the early 1980s, the nation experienced the spread of a cheap form of cocaine called "crack." Easy to produce and use (via smoking), this drug first emerged in a handful of American cities. By 1987, it was in forty-six states with users estimated to number between 4.2 and 5.8 million persons nationwide. The distribution of crack cocaine inside black communities produced black America's nefarious "crack epidemic."

A relatively cheap, but far more addictive substance than regular cocaine, crack is a crystal type of cocaine that is vaporized and inhaled by the user, producing an almost-immediate, intense, euphoric brain effect. Drug abuse studies revealed that addiction occurred much more rapidly with crack cocaine compared to heroin or other types of cocaine. Crack had dozens of cool slang names. It also had an alluring place in popular rap music and street talk that enticed unsuspecting youth and adults. However, crack ultimately destroyed the health of its users. Not only was it addictive, but the use of it over time increased the incidence of heart attacks, strokes, and psychiatric problems. Crack addiction also fueled risky social behavior, especially prostitution and unsafe sex. These practices greatly increased the risk of HIV infection, as well as other sexually transmitted diseases.

The crack problem was the primary impetus for the start of the national war on drugs. Political leaders, as well as police and drug control authorities, viewed crack as the most destructive substance of all among the nation's illicit drugs. Under the leadership of conservative political officials, a national "crime panic" arose over the fear of crack. Legislators and law enforcement authorities at all levels of government implemented rigorous criminal punishments for crack possession and distribution. Even crack-addicted pregnant women were subject to harsh punishment. Hospital emergency rooms began testing pregnant women for suspected cocaine use and reporting them to police authorities. By 1995, thirteen states had laws mandating that doctors report pregnant women or infants who tested positive for drug use to police. Some were imprisoned and in certain cases lost temporary or permanent custody of their children. In one Florida study in 1990, medical researchers found that among pregnant women addicts, regardless of whether the woman was examined at a public health clinic or in a private doctor's office, black women were ten times more frequently turned over to government health authorities compared to white pregnant women.

Government and drug policy planners paid little attention to the need for increasing preventive mental illness and rehabilitation resources, including job training and employment. This psychosocial approach could reduce the behavioral or psychological problems in vulnerable subgroups across the racial and class spectrum. However, the national social welfare and healthcare policymakers were unwilling or unable to address the psychosocial origins of the demand for crack. Consequently, the crack epidemic exploded across the nation.

Violent behavior and criminal incidents were endemic in neighborhoods in which trafficking of crack occurred. Urban communities trapped in New Ghetto conditions harbored pockets of crack users and sellers. Consequently, gun homicides and other violent crimes spilled out of black communities nationwide. Another health impact of crack involved prostitution. Addicted persons needing crack often turned to prostitution in exchange for the drug or money to purchase it. The combination of prostitution with IV and crack drug abuse increased cases of heterosexual transmissions of HIV. Thus the crack epidemic worsened the AIDS epidemic.

Between 1989 and 1993, AIDS cases among white males increased two and one-half times (from 17,500 to 43,600). For black males, the increase in AIDS over these four years was even steeper—from 8,000 to 28,500—some three and one-half times. Furthermore, black and Hispanic women experienced higher HIV rates compared to white women. In 1989, some 940 white females (thirteen years of age and over) were diagnosed with AIDS, compared to 1,900 black females. By 1993, the number of AIDS cases increased to 3,100 and 7,900 for these two female segments. Given the higher levels of HIV for black and Hispanic women, the threat of AIDS to black and Hispanic infants and children was greater, as well. In 1993, 60 percent of AIDS cases in children under the age of five were black, and 24 percent were Hispanic. In New York City, between 1990 and 1995, AIDS incidence grew by 56 percent among blacks, and 158 percent among heterosexual black women. At the same time, the street-level crack trade was making battle zones out of formerly tranquil neighborhoods.

For black Americans and New Activist health providers in particular, each rise in the number of heterosexual and child HIV cases in black communities heightened fears that the disease was spreading to the black community as a whole. Many blacks believed that AIDS was a form of racial genocide. They believed the federal government and white health scientists had conspired to somehow invent the virus and were bent on distributing it throughout black communities. The New Activists in the black medical care sector had to harness this growing popular anger. At the same time, both black healthcare and lay activists had to wrestle with behavioral realities within black communities. The incidents in which heterosexual infidelity resulted in HIV infections were particularly painful issues in black communities. Reports and stories of these new HIV victims began to appear in popular black media outlets.

One such 1991 story featured in *Ebony* magazine involved Denise K., a black middle-class mother of two daughters living in Atlanta, who discovered unexpectedly that she was HIV positive and that she had contracted the virus from her husband of seven years. Throughout Denise's marriage, her spouse had appeared to her as faithful, healthy, and non–drug addicted. However, when she tested positive for HIV, according to her interviewer, "she was flooded with an onslaught of emotions—self-pity, denial and hatred [toward her husband]." She was angry because "I got it [HIV] through heterosexual contact. I know I didn't do drugs. I didn't do anything else that could [have] caused me to get it. So that's where the hatred came in."[10]

The failure to protect black and other minority populations from the HIV epidemic left open a doorway for another overlapping epidemic: tuberculosis. While AIDS and crack had generated public outcries for solutions from throughout both black and mainstream America, the tuberculosis crisis was developing outside of national public and media attention. Beginning in the 1960s, with the spread of effective chemotherapies, isolation of infectious cases, and improved living conditions, tuberculosis rates had dramatically declined. However, throughout the late 1980s and 1990s, new cases of tuberculosis resurfaced, albeit rather quietly.

In 1987, the CDC reported nearly 23,000 tuberculosis cases in the nation. Whites comprised about one-half of these cases, while blacks made up some one-third, and Asian and Pacific Islanders and Native American and Alaskan Natives about one-tenth. Tuberculosis rates were especially growing in specific clusters of black and minority populations. New Ghetto living conditions lacked organized healthcare resources and adequate tuberculosis screening services. Populations living in such concentrated poverty were especially vulnerable to tuberculosis. In New York City, for example, new cases of tuberculosis grew from 1,307 in 1978 to 3,673 in 1991. Eighty percent of the tuberculosis cases were black or Latino, and one-quarter were homeless.

The new wave of tuberculosis in the 1980s and 1990s preyed especially upon people whose immune systems had already been weakened by HIV infection. With HIV rates already high in black American communities, when the nation experienced new tuberculosis outbreaks, the disease surfaced more widely in the black populations. Black populations also included subgroups of other persons located in high-risk physical spaces. These settings were conducive to close contact with persons possibly infected with tuberculosis—especially prisons, hospitals, cramped housing locations, and homeless shelters. There was also a strong link between tuberculosis cases and populations of IV drug users. As a result of all of these factors combined, tuberculosis rates began to spiral upward among the nation's black communities in the 1980s and 1990s.

The unique biology of the tuberculosis and HIV microbes reinforced simultaneous outbreaks of these two diseases. The different contagious qualities of the *M. tuberculosis* bacteria and the human immunodeficiency virus accounted for their tendency to coinfect the same individual. These different microbiological qualities of the HIV and tuberculosis agents also fueled the different paths and clusters of victims that surfaced within black communities. Consequently, wherever HIV epidemics have occurred, usually tuberculosis upsurges have been close behind, including those involving the more virulent strains of tuberculosis—so-called multidrug resistant tuberculosis (MDR-TB). Reported first in large hospitals and prisons in New York City, this form of tuberculosis was (and remains) particularly difficult to clinically treat. It is especially dangerous not only to immunocompromised populations but also to frontline healthcare providers as well.

Besides biological dynamics, the substandard and segregated housing as well as concentrated poverty in many black communities contributed to black America's high HIV and tuberculosis rates. While millions of middle-income blacks moved to the suburbs to escape the poverty of the New Ghetto, millions of low-income blacks did not, because they could not find affordable housing in the suburbs. One-fifth of the nation's blacks lived in what could be deemed a New Ghetto or, that is, concentrated poverty areas as of 1990, an increase of 36 percent from the number of blacks in such neighborhoods in 1980. Also, the number of black families living in poverty as defined by the federal government remained about the same from 1980 to the mid-1990s, roughly 31 percent. Whether living in visible New Ghettos or in adjacent multi-income city sections, the urban black population as a whole experienced greater black-white segregation compared to prior decades.

This complex social and cultural context was not the only factor that weighed against new epidemics dying down on their own. Many black residential areas lacked adequate health screening and primary care resources. This was the case not just in the black sections of major cities, but in the black suburban enclaves and rural districts, as well. Collectively, to the growing consternation of health advocates for black Americans, conditions in their communities provided a ripe setting for new tuberculosis and HIV infections.

The perils of New Ghetto urbanization, new disease epidemics, and a war on illicit drugs threw a dense fog over the equality vision—that is, the ideal that the health of blacks could one day equal that of whites. By the early 1990s, New Activists striving to improve health in black communities found themselves in neighborhoods gripped by illegal drug traffic and related gang and gun violence. These neighborhoods also had high concentrations of burned-out and abandoned houses, and youth unemployment rates as high as 30 to 60 percent!

With blacks experiencing new health perils and urban problems like AIDS and drug abuse, it was difficult to see how the historical struggle by blacks and their allies for the health equality ideal could progress. In the past, the black medical Achievers and Battlers had provided the leadership. However, this leadership was no longer cohesive and self-reliant, because the Black Medical World and the traditional black communities of preintegration America no longer existed.

In a study she coauthored with F. G. Murphy on diabetes in the black community, Joycelyn Elders, M.D., who, under President Bill Clinton, had served as the first African American U.S. surgeon general, addressed these difficult circumstances. They believed the community as a whole had to be mobilized to envision and execute healthcare solutions. In short, "community ownership, not reticence, must become the order of the day." Elders and Murphy recommended that this meant the vital first step for blacks was to somehow bring traditional cohesion back to the black community as a whole. Blacks needed to organize community "infrastructures" to take on the health problems in their communities. These infrastructures would incorporate not only medical professionals, but religious, political, educational, public safety, and business entities as well.[11] Elders and Murphy's call for community solidarity echoed the medical leadership of the Achievers and Battlers of old. However, the call by public health advocates alone was not enough to turn back the many "captains of death," from diabetes to AIDS, riding through urban black America in the last decade of the twentieth century. Still, the call combined with voices directly from victims and communities grew stronger, and so did self-reliant efforts to protect black collective health.

At the turn of the twenty-first century, broader social and environmental conditions shaped the medical disparities between blacks and other racial and ethnic groups. Moreover, natural disasters, industrial pollution, and epidemics would become increasingly important to address in efforts to realize the health equality ideal. Consequently, black Americans returned to self-reliance for guarding their health en masse. Many mobilized into local-, religious-, and culture-based community and social justice movements. These new movements centered on improving black health overall by attacking environmental injustices, the dangers of moral prejudice against disease victims, and the health policies that left out the poor and uninsured.

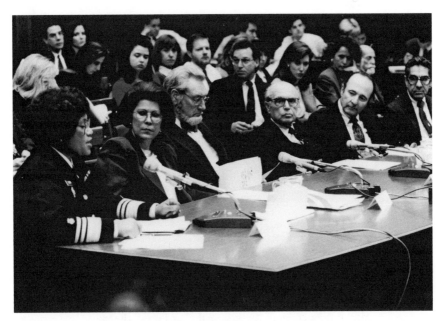

Figure 6.2.   Surgeon General Joycelyn Elders on a panel with former Surgeon Generals Antonia Novello and C. Everett Koop, ca. 1994.

Source: **National Library of Medicine.**

Chapter Seven

The AIDS Era and
the Time of Katrina

During the 1960s, 1970s, and early 1980s, there had been great strides in black health progress. The civil rights movement and the national response to urban riots had stimulated aggressive pro-welfare-state politics. This political change in turn led to a wide range of government-funded medical care and public health resources for black Americans and other racial and low-income minorities. However, in the last decades of the twentieth century, the struggle for black healthcare equality drifted into the shadows of national public issues. The operation of the nation's medical system became deeply enmeshed with financial, insurance, and political institutions. This development greatly fragmented social movements for healthcare equality, which simply were neither envisioned nor designed to wade into changing such complex administrative structures. After the late 1980s, it was not urban protests, or healthcare and civil rights organizations that shaped the nation's overall healthcare agenda. Instead it was the federal government and politicians who set it under constant pressure from free market-oriented hospital and medical service corporations, the private insurance sector, and competing public idealogues of morality.

During the presidencies of Ronald Reagan, George H. W. Bush, and William Clinton, other domestic policies fragmented the geography and economic viability of black communities even more directly. The federal government strove to meet private sector priorities such as suburbanization and expanding mass consumption markets more fully. In the area of urban housing, for example, in many cities, the government focused on reducing low-income housing (under Reagan) or placing such housing into private ownership (under Clinton).

As a result of the changes in the political and economic landscape in the 1980s and 1990s, the New Ghetto gradually spread, and so did inadequate healthcare for its residents. Many millions of black Americans, along with poorer Americans, found themselves without health insurance or physically unable to reach comprehensive hospital care. Instead these segments relied on emergency rooms, crowded public hospitals, or sporadic visits to solo physician practices. Whether in the Bronx, New York City; the South Side of Chicago; or the poor neighborhoods of Jackson, Mississippi—black healthcare advocates for these poor areas faced populations who were the embodiment of healthcare injustices. These residents and patients lacked prior health screenings and medical care, as well as lived in neighborhoods riddled with all forms of environmental pollution, social violence, and unsafe housing.

By the late 1980s, black healthcare advocates and their allied political and community groups were back to struggling locally against healthcare discrimination, this time with little fanfare in the national media. In the subsequent two decades, they faced the shift away from welfare-statism to full throttle Reaganomics and conservative New Liberalism. In the meantime, the nation's black health professionals remained largely woven into "safety net" medical institutions. Within this setting, many black physicians and other health professionals, as well as allied health workers and community leaders, stepped forward as New Activists. Each in his or her own way attempted to direct attention to the medical needs of black city, suburban, and rural communities. These health activists worked vigorously both within and against large health delivery institutions to shape programs and services appropriate for poorer black patients and black communities.

In the closing decades of the twentieth century, cities were experiencing multiple public health concerns. Among the most serious problems were the lack of resources adequate to roll back the spread of HIV, spikes in drug addiction, new tuberculosis cases, and high rates of chronic diseases linked to air pollution and poor nutrition. A new movement arose to address areas affected by "environmental racism," that is, whole inner-city neighborhoods with decades of built-up pollution in buildings, soil, water, and/or air from abandoned industrial and commercial sites as well as older, substandard housing. Most middle-income and more fortunate working-class segments of the population had been able to escape this inner-city housing and such commercial worksites, and move to the suburbs. Those left in these polluted neighborhoods were largely poor blacks and Latinos, with few options to remedy their situation.

However, since residential and social separatism concentrated blacks in specific housing tracts regardless of the diverse class characteristics of the black households, blacks of all social classes experienced common health problems, such as infectious diseases, at rates that were significantly higher compared to whites. In a Chicago study in 2000, journalists found that "despite [their] upward economic mobility [during] the prosperous latter half of the 1990s, members of the black middle class experience a radically different social reality than their white counterparts." The black middle class lived next to blocks "of blight, poverty, unemployment and crime." As one head of a local community development organization remarked, "For the middle class, it's hard to maintain the high lofty goals you have for yourself when this abject poverty is all around you."[1]

As the revenue base for the cities declined, so did their public hospitals, municipal services, and health-promoting policies such as building new affordable housing. The black health crisis—especially AIDS and deficient local medical resources—exploded at the same time as the flareup of drug abuse in the inner cities. As fallout from these crises spread, black healthcare leadership and community health activism reemerged. The struggle to develop self-reliant resources to promote black health has been the pattern for centuries. In earlier periods, black healthcare leaders had fought to keep slaves alive and facilitate their freedom; to deliver healthy babies in tenements and sharecropping communities; to keep the new urban families and workers of the Great Migrations healthy; to protect the health of veterans from two world wars; and to support the War on Poverty healthcare reforms. In the late twentieth century, this black leadership resurfaced once again—New Activism to face new challenges.

During the late 1980s and 1990s, the AIDS epidemic in black communities became the central issue in black health for both black America as well as the nation's medical establishment. Awareness of AIDS slowly expanded throughout black communities. However, each attempt at an organized initiative had to overcome strong undercurrents of racial suspicion, even paranoia about the problem. Based on a history of mistrust of white medical facilities and healthcare, many blacks believed both AIDS and the government's activities to eliminate the disease were actually a disguised strategy to commit black genocide. Some believed AIDS was the result of a plot by government laboratory scientists to devise a germ that would wipe out African people both on the continent of Africa and in the United States. Still others in the black public viewed AIDS as part and parcel of a broader genocide strategy of unleashing drug trafficking and gun violence, along with the AIDS epidemic, into America's black communities.

From the beginning of the AIDS epidemic, a cluster of black healthcare leaders or New Activists had emerged. These were medical and public health professionals, joined by other health workers and community organizers, who struggled to connect AIDS victims and at-risk groups, on one hand, and medical care services, government offices, and large charitable segments, on the other. To move partnerships forward, they had to overcome attitudes of alienation and mistrust widespread throughout vulnerable black communities, on one hand; and racial lethargy, confusion, and entrenched discrimination throughout the general public, on the other. These activists also had to break down the traditional walls that separated grassroots community groups and the large academic medical centers that were more interested in developing treatments and pharmaceutical aspects of HIV control. To influence the black public to discard conspiracy theories, the new black health advocates promoted commonsense knowledge and techniques known to prevent the transmission of AIDS and similar public health problems such as STDs.

One such New Activist was Dr. Louis W. Sullivan, among the most recognized and trusted black medical figures throughout the national black medical community. Among his many achievements, Sullivan eventually became the secretary of the Department of Health and Human Services under the George H. W. Bush administration. In 1993, when asked about racial-genocide conspiracy claims, he replied, "I've heard it and its poppycock, hogwash." Interviewed for a national black education publication, Sullivan emphasized that "AIDS has nothing to do with any kind of conspiracy or synthetic virus, the biology of Blacks[,] or their resistance or susceptibility."[2]

Little-known New Activists—doctors, nurses, caretakers, and community workers—worked throughout the New Ghetto city areas of the nation. Andrew D. McBride Jr (M.D., M.P.H.), health commissioner of Washington, DC, in the mid-1980s, appeared at numerous community and policy meetings to spread recognition of the critical health issues in inner-city black communities. Before AIDS in black communities became a national concern, McBride raised the awareness of his agency workers about appropriate treatment protocols and support for AIDS victims. In one 1986 incident, after an AIDS victim died in Washington, DC, his family members and friends waited in an adjoining room for six hours while city medical personnel refused to remove his body. McBride drove to the apartment building, entered, and covered and removed the body himself. He criticized the fears reflected in the media about such incidents. "The important lesson is not that the health commissioner went out to the scene, but the dramatization that AIDS is not transmitted through casual contact."[3]

Still, black public mistrust persisted as AIDS cases, and deaths, continued to rise throughout black America. Many black religious leaders and their congregants held to fundamentalist moral views, disdaining homosexuality and deeming it the core generator of the AIDS epidemic. Their explanations for and approaches to reducing AIDS clashed with those more secular community and public health activists who were intentionally nonjudgmental of persons and groups living with HIV. Some of the suspicion derived from memories of the Tuskegee Syphilis Study. Many black Americans referred to the study as the proof that the federal government had ill intentions with regard to the AIDS crisis in black communities. Another source of the suspicion was the reaction against prominent medical researchers and media sources announcing over and over that there was an "African" origin for the

AIDS virus and the AIDS epidemic as a whole. Many blacks, influenced by generations of Afrocentric research literature and religious beliefs, perceived these facts as blatantly false and simply white supremacist accusations against Africa.

These were rough years for black urban communities as they struggled against the AIDS and crack scourges. From the 1980s through the mid-1990s, many inner-city black neighborhoods were besieged by illegal drug traffic, gangs, and gun violence. These neighborhoods had large concentrations of burned-out housing and high youth unemployment rates that ranged from as high as 30 to 60 percent. Fear among white politicians and law enforcement authorities led to increased police force crackdowns and incarcerations, but little relief of the social conditions that spawned the drug use and related violence. Such actions reinforced conspiratorial attitudes among black city dwellers. Drawing on the ideas and writings of respected scholars and religious leaders, many surmised that AIDS, as well as crack, had been intentionally distributed in their communities to facilitate racial genocide.

Widely regarded black religious leaders contributed to the popularity of racial self-protection ideas and sentiments. Most notable among them was Minister Louis Farrakhan. He was and remains the highly influential leader of the Nation of Islam and the protégé of the religion's major founder, the Honorable Elijah Muhammad (1897–1975). Like Elijah Muhammad, Minister Farrakhan viewed white political leaders as masterminds behind social problems afflicting black communities, with the AIDS and crack epidemics just two of the most recent attempts to wipe out black America. Indeed, millions of black and Hispanic common folk believed that the drug trade in black and Hispanic communities had become a national priority only because the problem had been discovered in white communities.

Regardless of the widespread perception of conspiracies, the rank-and-file residents and social leaders in black communities had to somehow engage the AIDS epidemic. As the numbers of black AIDS-related deaths increased, many black community groups decided they needed to do something to help those in the late stages of AIDS. These victims were in need of living arrangements, medical assistance, spiritual counsel, and supportive hospital visits.

Many nonprofessional blacks and those in the human service fields had firsthand knowledge about the sufferings of blacks who had contracted AIDS, and placed only secondary importance on how the victim had contracted the disease in the first place. Moreover, interest in the need for community protection spread, as people feared the disease was spreading uncontrollably in the mainstream black adult population. By 1990, the NAACP's publication *The Crisis* carried articles about the AIDS crisis in black communities. In 1992, the NAACP board officially called attention to HIV/AIDS as a major public health crisis in the black American community.

The number of community projects to stem AIDS did, indeed, grow. However, there was some contention as to the best use of scarce health resources. Given the varied religious backgrounds and secular views as to why AIDS was striking blacks especially hard, black community leaders and neighborhood residents held widely conflicting stances on the best means to curtail the spread of HIV in their communities. Moreover, many viewed AIDS as just one of a multitude of life-and-death problems gripping black neighborhoods. They opposed HIV prevention measures if they believed these programs would intensify other social problems or take resources from the community's efforts to address these other problems. These leaders thought black communities should place a higher priority on eliminating drug abuse, teenage pregnancy and promiscuity, and street gangs.

One type of program that caused great controversy was the needle exchange program. In these programs IV drug users would be allowed to come off the streets into these centers and pick up clean syringes to administer their drugs to themselves. Health experts throughout the nation's leading AIDS organizations were certain needle-exchange programs were vital to cut down the spread of HIV among IV drug users. But many argued such programs did nothing to stop IV drug use and would even reinforce the acceptability of such behavior.

Initiatives to start clean-needle centers triggered vigorous divisions among blacks of all education and income levels, as well as political allegiances. Black religious fundamentalists and lay neighborhood leaders believed that once needle-exchange programs were set up in black neighborhoods, they would attract even more drug trafficking as well as tempt black children and youth to fall into drug abuse. Some with more conspiratorial viewpoints saw needle-exchange programs as designed to level the final blow to destroy black communities exactly by encouraging black drug use. For these reasons, needle-exchange programs were one such measure that many in black communities opposed.

In 1990, an outspoken black minister in Boston's Roxbury neighborhood, the Reverend Graylan Ellis-Hagler, aggressively opposed the establishment of a local needle-exchange program. He estimated some 2,500 recovering drug addicts lived within the reach of his ministry. When a group involved in drug abuse rehabilitation attempted to open a needle-exchange program, the minister, along with other activists from the neighborhood, picketed the site, and the police were forced to shut it down. According to Ellis-Hagler, white interests first "push drugs in the community," crippling it politically and economically. Next, "[t]hey send the males to jail. *Then* someone hands out needles to maintain the dependency. Meanwhile, grandmothers live in fear of their own children because of what white society made them become—crack addicts, throwaways."[4]

In spite of the early backlash against programs to lower the risk of AIDS in black neighborhoods, not all black church communities were so resistant to such initiatives. One by one, here and there, a black church started an activity or program to take on some aspect of the AIDS crisis. In 1985, Reverend Carl Bean and his Unity Fellowship Church in Los Angeles opened the Minority AIDS Project (MAP). This program provided comprehensive care for persons with AIDS. It also promoted education and essential health services to black and Latino communities in that city. It was the nation's first minority HIV/AIDS organization founded and operated by people of color. Other black ministers used their churches and nearby sister/brother churches to work with local health departments. In Baltimore, one such minister, Reverend Ben Jones of the New Psalmist Baptist Church, worked with the city health department and ten churches to educate their church members about the disease and the needs of AIDS victims.

Other community groups worked in partnership with black churches. The Black Leadership Commission on AIDS (BLCA) in metropolitan New York was one of the earliest large-scale community efforts to combat the AIDS epidemic. Founded in 1987, the organization developed into an information hub for over 750 black churches and more than 1,500 AIDS-related organizations. BLCA provided consultant support to black civic groups, clergy, and other professionals throughout the New York City area. By the early 1990s, it was working in partnership with the U.S. Centers for Disease Control and Prevention in various intervention programs.

African American immunologist and public health specialist Pernessa C. Seele exemplified the New Activists taking on the AIDS challenge. She realized that any efforts to fight the AIDS epidemic would have to include black churches. While she worked at the AIDS Initiative Program at Harlem Hospital in the 1980s, she was stunned by the lack of community support for the people and families suffering from AIDS. She found that the black community "neither understood the reasons for their pain, nor sought to alleviate their suffering." Seele asked, "How could Black America, for the first time in its history, turn away from brothers and sisters caught in a crisis that could destroy its community at its very roots? Why was the response to the AIDS crisis different from previous crises—enslavement, discrimination, and lynching?" She concluded that the missing factor was "the faith imperative—the directive from religious leaders to their congregations to learn, act and care as their Lord would expect of them in the age of HIV/AIDS."[5]

In 1989, Seele organized the first annual Harlem Week of Prayer, involving over fifty churches and mosques in programs that included AIDS awareness and prevention. After receiving funding from the Centers for Disease Control to start similar faith-based programming in other cities, Seele founded The Balm in Gilead, Inc., a nonprofit organization, to coordinate the efforts. The Black Church Week of Prayer for the Healing of AIDS started in six cities, with CDC funds for a pilot study, and grew annually in scope to become one of the largest such church-based projects. The Balm in Gilead has also gone on to partner with women's groups from the major African American denominations to create broader community health initiatives.

In 1993, the Balm in Gilead convened a weeklong National Education and Leadership Training Conference on AIDS, in Harlem, New York City. Jacquelyn Wilkerson, a leading church activist involved in AIDS issues and the interfaith religious community in Washington, DC, discussed the black church's resistance to join the anti-AIDS struggle in *Christian Century* magazine. She noted that the "traditional African-American religious community is very conservative in its views, [but] the one thing AIDS has done is to challenge our theology."[6] To ready black congregations to meet the challenge, Wilkerson joined with some five hundred other black clergy and laypeople for the weeklong conference.

In 1999, in conjunction with World AIDS Day and the tenth anniversary of the Black Church Week of Prayer for the Healing of AIDS, ministerial leaders of some of the nation's largest black churches gathered. They wanted to demonstrate that, in Seele's words, "[m]ore and more black religious leaders are sounding the call for greater attention to be paid to AIDS." These ministers and theologians agreed that they held strong, often differing positions on homosexuality, needle exchange, extramarital sex, and condom distribution. However, they agreed that "[a]nyone who knows anything about black people knows our churches . . . must lead us through the AIDS crisis." As the nationally popular Dallas minister and televangelist Rev. T. D. Jakes exclaimed, "Church, there is a way for us to do what needs to be done without violating what we believe."[7]

Other volunteer organizations not linked wholly with the church also emerged to take on AIDS at the community level. In 1985, Black and White Men Together founded a task force to help individuals and neighborhoods at high risk for AIDS in San Francisco. That same year, Blacks Educating Blacks about Sexual Health Issues, or Bebashi—Transition to Hope, formed in Philadelphia. Its goal was to provide assistance through street outreach to people with AIDS or at risk for the disease. Over the years it evolved into a multiservice health-service organization providing care for thousands of low-income blacks and other people of color with HIV and their families.

SisterLove, centered in Atlanta, also became one of the earliest and effective AIDS-control volunteer groups. It focused on educating black women about AIDS prevention and sexual health issues. Planning for SisterLove began in the late 1980s by its founder, Dazon Dixon Diallo, assisted by the women of color advisory board of the Women's AIDS Prevention Project. Officially incorporated in 1992, the organization grew into multifaceted programs. It trained volunteers to speak to audiences of students, mothers, young adults, gays, lesbians, and couples about safe sex practices. It also held workshops and participated in public events to increase awareness about the risks and realities of HIV/AIDS. Finally, it organized support groups for women living with HIV/AIDS to help them "to affirm themselves and experience spiritual, physical, mental and emotional healing."[8]

Churches and community organizations had come to the forefront in the struggle against AIDS. Likewise these institutions were vital to the New Activism that emerged in the fight against environmental pollution widespread in black communities. Substandard housing, air pollution, abandoned industrial buildings, and waste sites marred many of the nation's black neighborhoods and rural sections in this New Ghetto era. The flashpoint in the rise of environmental pollution as a major public health concern for black Americans had occurred in North Carolina during the 1970s and early 1980s. In Warren County, North Carolina, a largely poor, majority black county, black and white local residents took on the issue of a state-approved plan that would allow toxic waste to be dumped into their community. They were spurred on by church leaders with the United Church of Christ Commission for Racial Justice and activists with the NAACP. In 1973 a company involved in electrical transformers dumped a toxic material, polychlorinated biphenyl, or PCB, along the roadways of several North Carolina counties. The landfill site selected to house this contaminated soil was in the predominantly black town (Shocco) in Warren County, the state's county with the highest percentage of black residents.

Local ministers and other activists began direct protests against this plan decrying the proposed landfill as obvious race and class discrimination. Eventually national civil rights and environmental organizations joined with the protest movement. The NAACP pursued a major lawsuit on behalf of the protesting citizens of Warren County. The suit argued that the state of North Carolina had used funds from the U.S. Environmental Protection Agency in violation of Title VI of the U.S. Civil Rights Act, which prohibited federal funding of racially discriminatory public programs. Following multiple lawsuits, scientific surveys, and government hearings, in 1982 the state of North Carolina agreed with the county commissioners to curtail the landfill.

The Warren County controversy inspired other local public health, community, and religious grassroots organizations throughout the nation to take action against environmental racism. In numerous cities and town communities nationwide, these New Activist groups initiated protests, lawsuits, and other citizen actions against unfair conditions of pollution affecting poor and black communities. In response to the groundswell of public activism against environmental policy discrimination, the federal government, especially under the liberal administration of President Bill Clinton, developed innumerable measures on behalf of the idea of assisting citizens involved in environmental justice legal and political struggles.

Other environmental health struggles emerged involving black and poor communities that raised consciousness in both local and national healthcare and civil rights circles. These struggles illuminated the links between black health and behavioral problems such as excess cancers, asthma, and childhood disorders, on the one hand, and polluted environmental conditions that were major causes of these problems, on the other. In addition to toxic waste exposure, lead poisoning of children in poor minority communities surfaced as another critical public health danger in black communities. Beginning with little fanfare, in the mid-1970s public health researchers lead by Dr. Herbert Needleman presented research disclosing causal links between lead-poisoned children and serious learning and behavior disorders these children exhibited. As the years passed, public health experts, medical researchers, educators, and neighborhood groups, especially in large cities, joined forces to attack the lead poisoning hazard.

The health and community struggles against toxic lead pollution emerged most especially in pediatric care and educational institutions, housing improvement organizations, and child and youth social service agencies. Advocates from these various circles disclosed to government and public health authorities that hundreds of thousands of inner-city and rural children had absorbed unhealthy lead levels in their blood and organs. These children and their mothers had ingested this poisonous metal from eroding housing and school structures, playgrounds, contaminated drinking water, and baby food and liquids. In 1994, 90 percent of children living in New York City suffering from lead poisoning were black or Latino. Spurred by swelling numbers of public health conferences, epidemiological studies, and community protests, in the 1980s and 1990s, for the first time lead poisoning of the nation's black and poor children started gaining urgent attention in federal and local medical and children's agencies.

Indeed, issues such as toxic waste dumping in minority communities, as well as lead contamination in the living environments of inner-city and rural poor populations, set the stage for the critical takeoff of the environmental justice movement. In 1987, the United Church of Christ Commission for Racial Justice released its study exposing how toxic conditions were unfairly concentrated in black and minority residential areas. The survey, simply titled *Toxic Wastes and Race in the United States*, had an explosive national and international impact. Under the leadership of Reverend Ben Chavis, the Commission for Racial Justice publicized the study's findings at a press conference in Washington, DC. To many, this was the beginning point of what has become decades of incessant environmental justice struggles throughout America and the world.

The work by black community volunteer and religious sectors to combat the AIDS crisis and environmental injustice harkened back to the health campaigns during the time of the Black Medical World. In the early twentieth century, self-reliant black healthcare and civic groups and their white allies had played an important role in pushing forward the black healthcare agenda. National Negro Health Week, the black hospital movement, and the black public health nurses and black nursing organizations exemplified these self-reliant efforts. Now the anti-AIDS and the environmental justice movements were forcing black healthcare priorities onto the national public scene.

The Congressional Black Caucus (CBC) also became an important influence in making the fight against AIDS in black communities a national priority. For years the Caucus had come under growing criticism by concerned black community activists for essentially ignoring the AIDS crisis. Many black politicians just claimed they could not address AIDS because their districts were swamped with other urgent problems—especially illicit drugs, crime, and homelessness. However in 1992, pressure mounted, especially after the famous basketball player Earvin "Magic" Johnson publicly disclosed that he was HIV positive. In the months swirling around this national media event, the CBC joined directly in the AIDS fight. That year the Caucus protested the CDC's plan to cut some $14 million from dozens of groups that were operating AIDS projects in minority communities.

Some black Congress members solicited public testimony about the destructiveness of AIDS and prevention recommendations from victims and caregivers in their districts. In 1992, for example, Representative Donald M. Payne held congressional hearings on AIDS in his home state of New Jersey. The meetings addressed prevention, treatment, and education measures for combating AIDS. These efforts resulted in a larger allocation in the federal budget to help solve the AIDS crisis at various levels.

Other CBC members believed that some form of national health insurance or comprehensive coverage for all blacks and other minorities would meet the special medical needs of AIDS victims, but also victims of the black health crisis overall. In the major black business publication, *Black Enterprise* (May 1992), Representative Louis Stokes (D-Ohio) exclaimed that some thirty million Americans lacked health insurance, and an additional twenty million had insufficient health insurance. Therefore, it was "mandatory that we begin to try to give Americans—particularly minorities—adequate health care as a right."[9]

The average income for blacks as a whole reached historic highs during the Clinton years. Still even with this growing black middle class, many critical health problems in black communities intensified during the 1990s. President Clinton was moving toward reforming the nation's medical care delivery. His plan centered on putting healthcare delivery under a managed market model, as well as instituted government regulation of private health insurance providers. By contrast, many in the CBC stressed the need for a universal health insurance system. Representative John Conyers Jr., of Detroit, led both the CBC and the Democratic congressional groups in seeking a universal health insurance policy. Compared to mainstream politicians, black political and medical leaders overall believed that a national health insurance system was the only way to eliminate the black health crisis.

While most black Congress members favored government insurance that would cover all Americans, some prominent black medical professionals worked to promote President Clinton's comprehensive health reform initiative. In 1992, pediatrician and head of the Arkansas Department of Health Dr. Joycelyn Elders joined a national committee to advise the federal government on public health matters. In that capacity she worked to build support for the Clinton health reform plan. In early 1993, she was appointed surgeon general of the United States. Her association with Bill Clinton stemmed from his days as governor of Arkansas, and Dr. Elders had an established track record of accomplishments in improving the health of children, youth, and poor populations and communities.

In 1993, President Clinton introduced his plan, the Health Security Act, to Congress. While he shrewdly marketed his health proposal as a "universal coverage" plan that many mistook to mean a single-payer, national health insurance plan, in fact it was a so-called employer mandate plan. With a single-payer plan, one government unit pays for universal coverage and comprehensive benefits. This government unit also administers this national plan. The employer mandate plan requires employers provide health insurance to its employees and pay for all or part of the health insurance. In response, Conyers and some fifty Democratic congressional progressives called for a national health insurance system financed by the federal government. They intended for comprehensive national health insurance to correct fundamental limitations of the "managed competition" and employer mandate policy central to President Clinton's health plan. They believed that insurance companies, hospital associations, and drug companies profited the most from the existing system.

The progressive Democrats' bill would eliminate private health insurance and authorize the federal government to pay virtually all medical bills. This plan was to go in effect for all Americans within two years. In the end, both the Clinton health reform plan and the progressive plan were dashed by political opposition by the mid-1990s. The failure of both plans especially hurt blacks and other social segments that had large numbers of uninsured or underinsured persons. Throughout the 1990s, about one-fifth of the nation's blacks lacked health insurance. No matter how hard black politicians agitated for a national health plan, it was an unobtainable political goal given America's *realpolitik*, in which government essentially facilitated medical services through private health insurance–based financing. Even the huge federal programs like Medicaid and Medicare were organized more and more to flow within the private healthcare delivery structure. Increasingly hospitals and physicians were limited in the type and number of patients they treated by bureaucratic reimbursement systems established by government and health insurance regulators. These systems, rather than the physicians and medical specialists, also set the specifics of the clinical treatment received by patients.

Black doctors, like most others in their profession, were drawn into the larger mainstream medical sector—that is, healthcare delivery policies that were folding into the nation's expanding neoliberal economy. Neoliberal domestic policy is unlike the welfare-statism of the New Deal and Great Society eras. In a neoliberal social welfare agenda, while the government still tries to provide for social needs of the people, it does so by fostering the growth of markets and corporations to provide essential services and living needs such as healthcare, public education, and housing rather than having the government provide these vital resources directly.

By the 1990s and into the early twenty-first century, the general goal of the black physician's career had become assimilation into government agencies, mainstream medicine, and corporations. In 1998, NMA president Gary Dennis told his organization that the "promotion and support of alliances with corporate America and other medical associations such as the American Medical Association" were vital. These sectors, along with government agencies like the National Institutes of Health, he urged, could help them build "on our common goals and synergies that improve health care for our patients and promote the practice of medicine [as our] high priority."[10]

Despite the rise of the business sector as the managerial force of the nation's medical care system, New Activists still emerged. Many still remained involved even if indirectly with black-controlled institutions and community institutions. Some rose from the NMA and others from black health-related organizations and grassroots movements. These leaders realized that health equality for blacks, like national health insurance, was an ideal that had to be pursued if only incrementally. Like the Battlers and Bridge Builders, the New Activists sought small gains if necessary, which were rescue measures for the most desperately disadvantaged black Americans. These newest black health advocates strove to broaden the current medical safety net as well as grassroots institutions that, in turn, fostered stable black families and communities in those neighborhoods hardest hit by poverty, social violence, and governmental neglect.

Each city and rural county's safety net healthcare facilities and public health programs were vital for addressing the AIDS crisis and other immediate health problems in most black communities. These problems included excess numbers of blacks with undetected or untreated chronic diseases, especially cancer, heart disease, and diabetes; women's health issues, such as inadequate prenatal care, family planning services, and domestic abuse; and health problems of infants and children, such as insufficient vaccinations, asthma, homelessness, and lead-poisoning. Consequently, the NMA and other black health groups also advocated expanding government-funded medical coverage, especially Medicaid, to cover a larger population and requiring more employers to offer employee insurance.

While throughout the later 1990s, the NMA remained the national voice for black doctors, HMOs were siphoning patient populations from solo practitioners, including those of the black physicians in this sector. More than other racial or ethnic physician segments, black physicians in solo or small group practices treated a large proportion of black patients. However, in the marketplace model of medical care delivery that had taken hold, the "good old boy" network was resulting in HMOs that did not include these typical black physicians. Therefore, the NMA encouraged black health practitioners to unify into healthcare networks that could compete with those of the large insurance companies and HMOs.

NMA leaders also urged the government to support historically black medical schools, thus facilitating a sufficient supply of qualified black and minority health professionals. NMA president Tracy M. Walton Jr. had practiced for twenty-five years in a medically underserved section of Washington, DC. He spoke directly for black physicians and nurses in his 1994 speech in Virginia to the National Black Nurses Association (NBNA), when he said, "There must be a place for all of us who are health providers in any plans for reform. We [black physicians and nurses] have been the ones who took care of our people when nobody else would, could, or did. We are the ones who are now fighting to protect our community's interests."[11]

In addition, the NMA worked with other black health professionals and their organizations with direct links to black communities. It expanded its focus to mobilizing popular agencies that would address the full range of problems comprising the black health crisis, especially AIDS. To galvanize this process, the NMA first dealt with the professional obstacles facing practitioners within black communities or serving black patient constituencies. Like the Battlers of old, New Activists in the organization gave the clarion call to improve access to sufficient medical care for the nation's needy, poorer blacks.

In his speech to the NBNA, Dr. Walton urged the nation to take its head out of the sand. He implored everyone in America to spread the word about the nation's health crisis:

> I don't want to bore you or depress you with statistics, but wouldn't you say we were in a crisis when African Americans have higher mortality rates than whites for twelve of the fifteen major causes of death? Wouldn't you call it a crisis when the immunization rate from nonwhite children in the United States is lower than it is in fifty-five other countries? Wouldn't you call it a crisis when 20 percent of our people are uninsured, more than 25 percent are underinsured, and almost 30 percent get inadequate care?

Walton urged that both the black physicians' and nurses' organizations struggle in unison. Jointly, we show "we have a lot of power as a united community right now." He emphasized that "[t]ogether, as physicians and nurses, providers and patients, we can make a difference. For the sake of our people and ourselves, let's make healthcare reform our number-one priority."[12] In the 1990s, the NMA and NBNA worked with coalitions in fifteen cities as part of the U.S. Department of Health and Human Services' Healthy People 2000 program. Established in 1990, HP 2000 was a nationwide health promotion and disease prevention program with goals to strengthen the health of all Americans by the year 2000.

When inaugurated as the ninety-seventh president of the NMA in August 1998, Dr. Gary C. Dennis laid out challenges black America faced in the health arena. He said that his general focus would be eliminating disparities in healthcare. He characterized the HIV/AIDS epidemic as a threat to the very survival of the future black generations. This disease also was the number-one indicator of health disparities involving excessive, largely preventable disease and mortality rates. Dennis also noted that the rates of diabetes mellitus were 70 percent higher among African Americans and the prostate cancer rate among black men was 50 percent higher than that of whites.

Not all the racial disparities involving blacks compared to whites reflected negatively on black health. In 1998, David Satcher (M.D., M.P.H.) became the U.S. surgeon general. A black public health physician and former president of Meharry Medical College, Satcher had grown to exemplify the New Activist black medical leader. In his first year as surgeon general he issued a landmark survey on smoking and minorities in the United States. Smoking was associated with higher incidences of low-birth-weight infants, coronary heart disease, stroke, certain cancers, and specific respiratory diseases. The survey revealed that smoking among blacks, Hispanics, and other racial minorities had declined during the 1970s and 1980s in comparison to other minorities. Blacks had experienced the steepest decline of all the minorities. Despite such positive developments with regard to the health of blacks, gaps persisted for blacks in numerous health areas like chronic and infectious diseases, as well as in access to healthcare. In the 1990s, cigarette smoking rose substantially for both blacks and Hispanics.

The excessive AIDS rates for blacks and their lower access to healthcare resources remained the most significant racial disparity that carried over into the early 2000s. Blacks and Hispanics had experienced higher rates of heterosexual and IV drug use transmissions of HIV in the first years of the epidemic, as well as high rates of transmission among populations in risky settings such as prisons. These rates predictably indicated that AIDS incidence would rise among black women and in settings where IV drug users or transient populations were heavily concentrated.

Indeed, in the mid-1990s, black women in the South began exhibiting the highest rates of HIV infection among American women. This trend continued in 2000 and beyond. For example, the percentage of black women among newly reported HIV patients in Alabama grew from 13 percent in 1990 to 31 percent in 2000. In North Carolina during the same period, black women went from 18 to 27 percent of the state's HIV-infected population. Black women comprised about one-third of newly reported cases in Mississippi in 2000. Between 1999 and 2002 the CDC amassed data for twenty-nine states and "discovered" that blacks (some twenty-seven thousand) accounted for three-fourths of the nation's HIV cases that had been acquired through heterosexual contact.

In another investigation in 2001, the *New York Times* reported that "in many ways AIDS in the South is more like AIDS in the developing world than in the rest of the United States." Joblessness, poor education, minimal access to healthcare, and dismal social outlooks among the South's poor produced undetected HIV cases. This report emphasized that among black women in the South living in poverty, there was a widespread feeling of powerlessness about HIV risks. "All of their life experiences teach them that they have very little control over their futures. [They] sense you don't control your life that much, and if God wants me to have HIV, I'll get it."[13]

Despite strong initiatives by black medical organizations as well as numerous black religious and civic organizations across the nation to come to grip with AIDS, in the late 1990s there were definite continuing divisions between black health leaders and politicians, on one hand, and the more insulated views of mainstream medical organizations and health policymakers, on the other. Many national authorities took the position that AIDS was declining as a national crisis. They pointed to the fact that the death rate for AIDS had been falling nationwide. By contrast, black health professionals and political activists cried out that AIDS was an urgent issue and symbolic of an entire range of black health crises.

Moreover, medical research on AIDS had progressed steadily. Clinical researchers were increasingly optimistic about developing treatments for AIDS in the near future. Their confidence stemmed from a growing body of clinical data revealing that HIV infection could be constrained when combination antiretroviral drug therapy was used early in the infection process. Incorporated into a clinical treatment approach known as HAART (highly active antiretroviral therapy), these drugs blocked the replication of the human immunodeficiency virus in the peripheral blood and tissue reservoirs. As a consequence, these drugs countered the intensification of HIV infection in individuals, enabling a growing number of persons with HIV and AIDS to live healthier and longer than in the early years of the epidemic. Antiretroviral drugs also reduced HIV secretions associated with sex that, in turn, substantially lowered the risk of sexual transmission. As leading biomedical researcher David Ho stated in 1997, "the overall picture at the moment is that we can control the virus well, and we can have an impact on the disease [in individuals] for prolonged periods of time."[14]

Nonetheless, black leadership scrutinized the declining national rates of AIDS cases that began in 1993 in a fundamentally different way, emphasizing that AIDS still remained the leading cause of death for blacks between the ages of twenty-five and forty-four. As of 1998, nearly one-half of the nation's AIDS deaths were black, and one-fifth were Hispanic. That year Surgeon General Satcher told the press, "I don't think there is any question that [AIDS] in this country is becoming increasingly an epidemic of color."[15]

Regardless of the opposing camps about whether or not AIDS was an urgent threat—between blacks and whites, as well as between segments within the black community—most blacks supported efforts to take on the AIDS battle as a top political priority. The AIDS crisis was simply too intense for any sector of black political leadership or civil rights activism to ignore. While many AIDS healthcare and research programs focused on finding new drug regimens to treat persons with HIV, black and Latino organizations focused on prevention programs in the community setting that could reduce the spread of HIV and the disease in the first place. Their programs were so effective that leading mainstream AIDS organizations began adding black and Latino organizers to their leadership, hoping to learn from them. In the meantime, federal officials in charge of Medicaid got in step by improving rules for AIDS patients on Medicaid. These recipients could now receive their coverage sooner in their illness, as opposed to having to wait until they had developed full-blown AIDS.

Kweisi Mfume, the president of the NAACP, led that organization toward more supportive work in the fight against AIDS, joining the board of the National Black Leadership Commission on AIDS. The CBC leadership also pressed President Clinton into passing into action a $156 million bill that focused on AIDS prevention programs specifically targeted for minorities. This allocation rose to $245.4 million the following year. With the emergence of significant funds, many new programs and services to attack the AIDS problem in black communities at the neighborhood and interpersonal level developed. Positive results in the battle against AIDS followed as the years of struggle continued.

In 2000, black religious and political AIDS activists joined a nationwide gospel campaign called ONE VOICE. The aim of the project was to expand public awareness on a national scale about the HIV/AIDS crisis. In a series of events organized with the CBC and Surgeon General David Satcher, famous gospel music artists such as Vickie Winans, Edwin Hawkins, Sandra Crouch and Andraé Crouch, and Kirk Franklin held concerts in major U.S. cities. The concerts were to promote AIDS education and volunteer HIV testing throughout black communities. Other key organizers included the Reverend

Yvette Flunder as well as Bobby Jones, the host of a legendary gospel television show on the Black Entertainment Network, and basketball star Earvin "Magic" Johnson.

At the end of the 1990s, the black "health crisis" was far from over. However, the term was being increasingly replaced by "black health disparities" in policy circles and public discourse. In earlier decades the phrase "black health crisis" was used primarily to describe health conditions and lack of access to healthcare in poor black communities. By the close of the 1990s, public health and medical authorities, as well as political leaders, were more focused on the clinical dimensions of black health problems. The digital culture emerged and amplified the popular circulation of the "health disparities" term now favored by medical and policy circles.

Between 1999 and 2002, the National Academy of Sciences' Institute of Medicine surveyed the health disparities of black Americans and other racial minorities. Its 2003 report, *Unequal Treatment: Confronting Racial and Ethnic Disparities in Health Care,* found that, in general, black patients still did not receive the same level of effective care as did whites. Health status indicators were substantially lower for blacks in comparison to whites. These racial disparities prevailed even when black and white patients had similar socioeconomic, age, and health insurance characteristics. Moreover, when treating blacks for major diseases such as cancer, heart disease, and HIV/AIDS, doctors applied fewer treatment options conventionally recommended by the medical specialities.

The report urged the entire nation to seek broader awareness of the disparities. As for medical institutions, it recommended that they follow "evidence-based" guidelines in making decisions about treatment and coverage plans. Finally, the report stressed the need to expand the supply of minority health providers, since these caregivers were more likely to work with minority populations and communities. As the Institute emphasized, the main way to eliminate racial disparities in health was to streamline the healthcare system according to the best scientific evidence available.

Other studies also noted the need to improve the supply of blacks and minorities in the health professions. The number of black medical professionals had been flat from the 1980s all the way through the 1990s. By 2004, black doctors were only between 3 and 4 percent of the nation's physician supply. The W. K. Kellogg Foundation sponsored the Louis Sullivan Commission on Diversity in the Healthcare Workforce to gather facts from a wide range of health, community, and business leaders on the issue of black and minority underrepresentation in the medical fields. In its major report, *Missing Persons: Minorities in the Health Professions* (2004), the Commission recommended numerous ways to increase the supply of black and minority health professionals. It also stressed that a pivotal value in the health professions must be diversity. But while government experts and foundations strove to curtail racial disparities in the medical resources and treatment pipeline for the most needy black communities and populations, racial discrimination built into the larger medical system proved extremely difficult to eliminate.

In 2005, Hurricane Katrina exposed the profound weaknesses of urban "safey net" healthcare. The black, Creole, and multicultural communities of New Orleans have been the fountainhead for America's jazz and "root" culture heritage. Just before Katrina struck, about two-thirds of the city's population was African American. Even though traditionally about one-fourth of modern New Orleans citizens were economically poor, the dynamic musical culture of its African American and Creole community populations always shone through, not only to the nation but to the world. Katrina all but destroyed many of these communities. It leveled or damaged two-thirds of the city's housing—some 134,000 housing units. One year after the storm, only 209,000 of the city's pre-hurricane population of 455,000 residents had returned. By 2010, the city's population of 344,00 was about three-fourths its pre-Katrina level. Many blacks who did not return to New Orleans simply could not afford to. In other cases, they had lived in neighborhoods that had been totally devastated and that authorities never rebuilt. Thus, there was no house or community to return to.

Even before Hurricane Katrina, many among the New Orleans black population were unhealthy, and uninsured, as well. Blacks faced high levels of infant mortality, as well as chronic diseases like diabetes and heart disease, asthma, and AIDS. For these health categories, blacks in the city and in Louisiana had some of the highest rates in the nation. Medical resources in New Orleans prior to the hurricane were seriously deficient. In the few months following the storm, the core section of New Orleans (Orleans Parish), nearly one-third of the residents relied on Medicaid for health insurance.

While the storm and flooding diminished health and medical care for hundreds of thousands of persons in New Orleans and in the larger Gulf region, this chaotic event amplified in particular the structured or fixed inequality of healthcare resources that low-income populations faced. When Katrina struck, New Orleans had two major hospitals operated by Louisiana State University's Medical Center—Charity Hospital and University Hospital. Of the two, Charity Hospital had been the center for hospital care for the city's poor people of color. Prior to Katrina, almost three-quarters of its patients were blacks, most with incomes below $20,000. In 2003, over half of Charity's patients lacked health insurance, compared to just 4 percent for the city's other hospitals. Before Katrina, Charity provided sorely needed care for HIV/AIDS, drug abuse, and psychiatric as well as trauma care. Charity also was a major center for training and employing thousands of the city's and state's nurses, physicians, and other health professionals. Damage to both hospitals was extensive, but only University Hospital reopened and this more than a year after Katrina.

With the city's health system and police force having to rebuild from shambles, health as a minimal right to physical security was not available to New Orleans residents for many years after the storm. Violent crimes flared up, becoming a major impediment to communities recovering from the storm damage. At the end of 2006, the homicide rate in New Orleans was about 20 percent higher than that of any other city in the nation. Desperately needed mental health and drug treatment facilities were also heavily damaged by the hurricane, contributing to the high crime rate. Before the hurricane, University Hospital was a 575-bed facility with multiple departments, including psychiatric services, but by 2009, after extensive renovations, it operated solely as a trauma care facility to fill the city's urgent need for emergency care services.

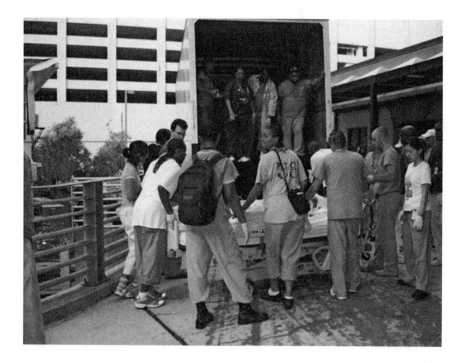

Figure 7.1.   Patients evacuated at the New Orleans Veterans' Affairs Medical Center, New Orleans, Louisiana (2005), during the Hurricane Katrina catastrophe. All patients were relocated safely.

Source: **U.S. Department of Veterans' Affairs, Southeast Louisiana Veterans' Health Care System, "VA New Orleans 'The Legacy of Service' Continues," accessed August 31, 2017, at https://www.neworleans.va.gov/Legacy_of_service.asp.**

The federal government directed billions of dollars to post-Katrina New Orleans to build or repair bridges, schools, and streets. Still, economic poverty linked with racial discrimination returned in full force to New Orleans and the Gulf Coast. By 2010, the poverty level for the city had returned to its highest rate since 1999. Forty-two percent of the city's children were living in poverty, as was 27 percent of the city's overall population. Among the city's skyrocketing poverty rates, 34 percent of New Orleans blacks were in poverty, compared to 14 percent of whites. A stunning 65 percent of black children under the age of five lived in poverty, compared to under 1 percent of white children.

In the years following Hurricane Katrina, black health disparities remained widespread as well. Between 2008 and 2010, blacks in New Orleans were three times more likely to die of diabetes compared to whites. The death rate for blacks from kidney disease and HIV were double those of whites. Black youth in New Orleans (aged eighteen to twenty-four) were four times more likely to die from any cause compared to white youth of the same age. In 2010, major chronic disease risks for blacks such as hypertension and high blood pressure, as well as asthma, were roughly double that of white residents.

Finally, from 2009 to 2011, almost one-third of the black residents of New Orleans aged eighteen to sixty-four lacked health insurance, compared to 17 percent of whites. Writing in a Louisiana publication on multicultural issues, local policy analyst Lance Hill asked his city and the larger public not to deny disparities. "With all the triumphal rhetoric of New Orleans as a city rising from the dead," he stated, health data "offers the harsh truth that some have risen while others have fallen. We act at our own peril if we ignore these troubling developments."[16]

Unlike in the Civil Rights Era, during the critical years of the AIDS and Katrina crises, New Activists in the black health and civil rights organizations had not found a way to make black health equality a specific and urgent priority to the federal government and medical policymakers. A symptom of this national lethargy has been the number of black Americans enrolled in the nation's medical schools, which has not improved between 1978 and 2014. Indeed, there were fewer black men in U.S. medical schools in 2014 than in 1978.

In the years immediately following the Hurricane Katrina catastrophe, the nation's political leaders and health policymakers soul-searched deeply for ways to repair the healthcare delivery system—a system that had obviously marginalized millions of America's uninsured, poverty-stricken, and financially pressed middle class. When Senator Barack Obama swept into the presidency in 2008, a centerpiece of his administration became the Patient Protection and Affordable Care Act (ACA), or so-called Obamacare, passed in 2010.

The ACA greatly reduced the number of uninsured Americans from about 49.9 million in 2010 to 30 million in 2016. Among the newly insured, between 2013 and 2016 some three million blacks and four million Latino Americans previously uninsured obtained insurance. The ACA expanded civil rights legal protections to gender minorities by banning federal funds to any health entity that discriminated on the basis of gender orientation. The law also prohibited insurance companies from denying coverage to citizens with preexisting conditions. Thus, as of 2016 the ACA protected about 129 million persons who had some type of preexisting physical condition. The eligibility requirements for Medicaid were also changed by the ACA. Medicaid now included all adults with incomes below 133 percent of the federal poverty level. This provided Medicaid coverage to an estimated 4.4 million additional adults.

The environmental justice and anti-AIDS movements, as well as the Katrina catastrophe, had shed light on the quiet yet devastating vulnerability that the poor and ill among blacks and other minorities experienced. The economic and political priorities that had shaped America's cities and suburbs since the 1970s had also shaped the unequally distributed, highly expensive medical system. In the end, even as the health reforms of the Obama administration unfolded, the medical system nonetheless still operated with gaping holes. Many millions of poor persons of color and others lacking financial means and access to quality healthcare—these were the citizens falling into the holes the health reforms could not fill. Despite progress, the country still has further to go to achieve the health equality ideal fully.

We first began this story during the American Revolution and Civil War eras. African Americans and abolitionists in the healing arts, conjurers, and midwives strove to protect life itself for the slaves and freed blacks of America. This same struggle—caretakers attempting to save black people from threats to their health due to material poverty and color—took place again and again—from the Achievers of the Nadir and Jim Crow periods; to the Battlers and Bridge Builders of the Civil Rights and Urban Crisis periods; to the New Activists of the present. In the last few decades, the struggle for health and care has been waged inside postindustrial cities, and the black and Latino enclaves of metropolitan suburbs. But it is the same old struggle: to achieve equality in healthcare.

In New Orleans, on the tenth anniversary of Hurricane Katrina, August 29, 2015, the city's people staged hundreds of events in remembrance of the 1,800 residents who lost their lives in the storm. Public community and musical activities, as well as gatherings of family, friends, and neighbors—each celebrated surviving a decade of post-Katrina challenges. Many of the events focused on wellness programs, health screenings, and interfaith support. The drive to make the city a community that cares for health equality was as strong as ever.

Selected Bibliography

For general histories of the medical experience of African-Americans, the essential sources are Herbert M. Morais, *The History of the Negro in Medicine* (1968); and W. Michael Byrd and Linda A. Clayton, *An American Health Dilemma: Race, Medicine, and Health Care in the United States, 1900–2000* (2 volumes; 2002). Morais's classic book gives a starting point to the full spectrum of black medical achievements and professional struggles through the Civil Rights Era. Byrd and Clayton's *American Health Dilemma* is exhaustive in range and centered on its key thesis that an apartheidlike racial caste underlies American medical care. On the modern black medical experience focusing on policies and financing, see David B. Smith, *Health Care Divided: Race and Healing a Nation* (1999). For a history of the scientific exploitation of blacks by the medical profession, see Harriet A. Washington, *Medical Apartheid: The Dark History of Medical Experimentation on Black Americans from Colonial Times to the Present* (2006).

For the physical health of African American slaves and their living conditions on the plantations, see Todd L. Savitt, *Medicine and Slavery: The Care of Blacks in Antebellum Virginia* (1978; reprint 2002). The general histories above also cover slavery, the Civil War, and Reconstruction black health issues. On the demography and epidemiology of enslaved Africans and American-born slave populations throughout the colonies and early United States, see Kenneth F. Kiple and Virginia Himmelsteib King, *Another Dimension to the Black Diaspora: Diet, Disease, and Racism* (1981); Kenneth F. Kiple (ed.), *The African Exchange: Toward a Biological History of Black People* (1987); and the articles in Paul Finkelman's edited volume, *Medicine, Nutrition, Demography, and Slavery* (1989).

On the health of women slaves, see Sharla M. Fett, *Working Cures: Healing, Health, and Power on Southern Slave Plantations* (2002); and Marie Jenkins Schwartz, *Birthing a Slave: Motherhood and Medicine in the Antebellum South* (2006). For indigenous health practices based on narratives of ex-slaves, see Herbert C. Covey, *African American Slave Medicine: Herbal and Non-Herbal Treatments* (2007).

The fine-grain history of black American health in the tumultuous Civil War–Reconstruction Period has grown. See Margaret Humphreys, *Intensely Human: The Health of the Black Soldier in the American Civil War* (2008); Jim Downs, *Sick from Freedom: African-American Illness and Suffering during the Civil War and Reconstruction* (2012); and Gretchen Long, *Doctoring Freedom: The Politics of African American Medical Care in Slavery and Emancipation* (2016).

The so-called Nadir period in the late nineteenth and early twentieth centuries saw harsh poverty and segregated health care conditions throughout the South. On biological determinism, the idea that blacks were an inherently weaker race compared to whites, and its influence on black health care, see Vanessa Northington Gamble, *Germs Have No Color Lines: Blacks and American Medicine, 1900–1940* (1989); David McBride, *From TB to AIDS: Epidemics among Urban Blacks since 1900* (1991); and Samuel K. Roberts Jr., *Infectious Fear: Politics, Disease, and the Health Effects of Segregation* (2009). The impact of public water and sewage systems on black Southern health is covered in Werner Troesken, *Water, Race, and Disease* (2004). On the inadequate healthcare and social conditions of the South's black and white working classes in this period, see Edward H. Beardsley, A *History of Neglect: Health Care for Blacks and Mill Workers in the Twentieth-Century South* (1987). The policies and politics of Southern healthcare segregation are covered by Karen Kruse Thomas, *Deluxe Jim Crow: Civil Rights and American Health Policy, 1935–1954* (2011).

Black healthcare networks and medical training institutions were vital to black communities during the Jim Crow decades. On black medical schools, see Todd L. Savitt, *Race and Medicine in Nineteenth- and Early Twentieth-Century America* (2007); James L. Curtis, *Blacks, Medical Schools, and Society* (1971); and James Summerville, *Educating Black Doctors: A History of Meharry Medical College* (1983). On the background, professional lives, and social leadership of black physicians in the Jim Crow South, see Thomas J. Ward Jr., *Black Physicians in the Jim Crow South* (2003). The nursing professions are covered by Darlene Clark Hine, *Black Women in White: Racial Conflict and Cooperation in the Nursing Profession, 1890–1950* (1989); Althea T. Davis, *Early Black American Leaders in Nursing: Architects for Integration and Equality* (1999); and Phoebe Pollitt, *African American and Cherokee Nurses in Appalachia: A History, 1900–1965* (2016).

Throughout the first half of the twentieth century, black medical activists and social welfare leaders consistently organized public health projects in poor black communities. Histories of such community health projects, and the black professionals and activists who mobilized them, can be found in Susan Smith, *Sick and Tired of Being Sick and Tired: Black Women's Health Activism in America, 1890–1950* (1995); Diane Kiesel, *She Can Bring Us Home: Dr. Dorothy Boulding Ferebee, Civil Rights Pioneer* (2015); and David McBride, *From TB to AIDS: Epidemics among Urban Blacks since 1900* (1991).

Traditional health practitioners and folk beliefs were widespread throughout the black South and, to a lesser extent, the black North during the first two-thirds of the twentieth century. For this history, see Margaret Charles Smith, *Listen to Me Good: The Life Story of an Alabama Midwife* (1996); Onnie Lee Logan, *Motherwit: An Alabama Midwife's Story* (1991); Sharon A. Robinson, "A Historical Development of Midwifery in the Black Community," *Journal of Nurse-Midwifery* 29 (1984): 247–50; and Wilbur H. Watson, *Black Folk Medicine: The Therapeutic Significance of Faith and Trust* (1984).

On black hospitals in the pre–*Brown vs. the Board of Education* and civil rights periods, Vanessa Northington Gamble has written a number of valuable works: *Making a Place for Ourselves: The Black Hospital Movement, 1920–1945* (1995); "The Provident Hospital Project: An Experiment in Race Relations and Medical Education," *Bulletin of the History of Medicine* 65 (1991): 457–75; and *The Black Community Hospital: Contemporary Dilemmas in Historical Perspective* (1989). Other important historical studies include Thomas Holt, Cassandra Smith-Parker, and Roselyn Terborg-Penn, *A Special Mission: The Story of Freedmen's Hospital* (1975); Mitchel F. Rice and Woodrow Jones Jr., *Public Policy and the Black Hospital: From Slavery to Segregation to Integration* (1994); and David T. Beito, "Black Fraternal Hospitals in the Mississippi Delta, 1942–1967," *Journal of Southern History* 65 (1999): 109–40. On the large public hospitals that heroically served the black poor and other disadvantaged city populations, see Aubre de L. Maynard, *Surgeons to the Poor: The Harlem Hospital Story* (1978); Harry F. Dowling, *City Hospitals: The Undercare of the Underprivileged* (1982); and David Ansell, *County: Life, Death, and Politics at Chicago's Public Hospital* (2011).

The history of blacks in dentistry can be garnered from the following works: Clifton O. Dummett, *The Growth and Development of the Negro in Dentistry in the United States* (1952); H. H. Haynes, "An Historical Perspective of Blacks in American Dentistry," *Dental School Quarterly* 5 (1989): 5–8; J. M. Hyson Jr., "African-American Dentists in the United States Army: The Origins," *Journal of the Massachusetts Dental Society* 44 (1995): 23–26; C. O. Dummett and L. D. Dummett, "A Retrospective of America's Second National Dental Association," *Journal of the American College of Dentistry,*" 70 (2003): 18–25; Clifton O. Dummett, "National Museum of Dentistry

Exhibition: The Future Is Now! African-Americans in Dentistry," *Journal of the National Medical Association* 95 (2003): 879–83; J. W. Jamerson, "A Sterling Legacy," *Journal of Health Care for the Poor and Underserved* 19 (2008): 1–9; and Elizabeth Mertz, J. Calvo, C. Wides, and P. Gates, "The Black Dentist Workforce in the United States," *Journal of Public Health Dentistry* 77 (2017): 136–47.

The general histories mentioned in the first paragraph all cover the impact of the civil rights movement on the struggle for black equality in medical care and health conditions. There are important specialized histories that deal with specific health policies, hospitals, medical schools, and the various medical professions. See Dietrich C. Reitzes, *Negroes and Medicine* (1958); and David McBride, *Integrating the City of Medicine: Blacks in Philadelphia Health Care, 1910–1965* (1989). On physicians mobilizing and contributing to the civil rights movement, see John Dittmer, *The Good Doctors: The Medical Committee for Human Rights and the Struggle for Social Justice in Health Care* (2010). On grassroots community responses to the medical discrimination of this period, see Alondra Nelson, *Body and Soul: The Black Panther Party and the Fight against Medical Discrimination* (2013); and Jenna Loyd, *Health Rights Are Civil Rights: Peace and Justice Activism, 1963–1978* (2014).

In the 1960s and 1970s, black populations compared to whites had higher levels of chronic diseases such as certain cancers and diabetes. Valuable historical studies of these subjects include Keith Wailoo, *How Cancer Crossed the Color Line* (2011) and *Dying in the City of the Blues: Sickle Cell Anemia and the Politics of Health and Race* (2001). For a groundbreaking public health history of Southern blacks and sexually transmitted diseases, see James H. Jones, *Bad Blood: The Tuskegee Syphilis Experiment* (1981; 1993). For an anthology of medical studies valuable for discerning the history of black health problems in the 1960s and 1970s, see Richard A. William, *Textbook of Black-Related Diseases* (1975). On mental illness, see Audrey Thomas and Samuel Sillen (Introduction by Kenneth B. Clark), *Racism and Psychiatry* (1972); and Jonathan M. Metzl, *The Protest Psychosis: How Schizophrenia Became a Black Disease* (2009).

For the history of the black health crisis of the 1980s and early 1990s, see R. L. Braithwaite and Sandra E. Taylor (eds.), *Black Health Issues in the Black Community* (1992); and Laurie K. Abraham, *Mama Might Be Better Off Dead: The Failure of Health Care in Urban America* (1993). Sources important for public health and policy history can be found in Mitchell F. Rice and Woodrow Jones Jr., *Black American Health: An Annotated Bibliography* (1987). On black women's health priorities during this period, see Evelyn C. White (ed.), *The Black Women's Health Book: Speaking for Ourselves* (1990; 1994 expanded edition); and Dorothy Roberts, *Killing the Black Body: Race, Reproduction, and the Meaning of Liberty* (1998). On the persistent legacy of the Tuskegee Syphilis Study through the 1990s, see Susan M. Reverby, *Tuskegee's Truths: Rethinking the Tuskegee Syphilis Study* (2000); and Ralph V. Katz and Rueben Warren (eds.), *The Search for the Legacy of the USPHS Syphilis Study at Tuskegee: Reflective Essays Based upon Findings from the Tuskegee Legacy Project* (2013).

On the unionization of black hospital workers along with other minority and working-class hospital labor, see Karen Sacks, *Caring by the Hour: Women, Work, and Organizing at Duke Medical Center* (1987); and Leon Fink and Brian Greenberg, *Upheaval in the Quiet Zone: A History of Hospital Workers' Union, Local 1199* (1989) and second edition, *Upheaval in the Quiet Zone: 1199SEIU and the Politics of Health Care Unionism* (2009).

For an historical study of blacks and the AIDS crisis, see Harlon L. Dalton, "AIDS in Blackface," in *The AIDS Reader: Social, Political, Ethical Issues*, ed. by Nancy F. McKenzie (1991), 122–43; David McBride, *From TB to AIDS: Epidemics among Urban Blacks since 1900* (1991); Cathy Cohen, *The Boundaries of Blackness: AIDS and the Breakdown of Black Politics* (1999); Jacob Levenson, *The Secret Epidemic: The Story of AIDS and Black America* (2004); and Sonja Mackenzie, *Structural Intimacies: Sexual Stories in the Black AIDS Epidemic* (2013). For an overview of health disparities and formation of the Affordable Care Act or so-called Obamacare, see Toni P. Miles, *Health Care Reform and Disparities: History, Hype, and Hope* (2012).

Biographies and autobiographies of both prominent and lesser-known black physicians provide vivid descriptions of the periods and themes this book has covered. Noteworthy among such works are: James P. Comer, M.D., *Beyond Black and White* (1972); Charles E. Wynes, *Charles Richard Drew: The Man and the Myth* (1988); Spencie Love, *One Blood: The Death and Resurrection of Charles R. Drew* (1996); Yvonne S. Thorton, *The Ditchdigger's Daughter* (1995); Ben Carson, with Cecil Murphey, *Gifted Hands: The Ben Carson Story* (1990); Joycelyn Elders, M.D., *From Sharecropper's Daughter to Surgeon General of the United States* (1998); Sara Lawrence-Lightfoot, *Balm in Gilead: Journey of a Healer* (1995); Gilbert R. Mason, M.D., with James Patterson Smith, *Beaches, Blood, and Ballots: A Black Doctor's Civil Rights Struggle* (2000); Hugh Pearson, *Under the Knife: How a Wealthy Negro Surgeon Wielded Power in the Jim Crow South* (2000); Carl C. Bell, M.D., *The Sanity of Survival: Reflections on Community Mental Health and Wellness* (2004); and Louis W. Sullivan, with David Chanoff, *Breaking Ground: My Life in Medicine* (2014).

On the environmental justice movement, see United Church of Christ Commission for Racial Justice, *Toxic Wastes and Race: A National Report on the Racial and Socio-Economic Characteristics of Communities with Hazardous Waste Sites* (1987); Robert D. Bullard, *Dumping in Dixie: Race, Class, and Environmental Quality* (2000); Eileen McGurty, *Transforming*

Environmentalism: Warren County, PCBs, and the Origins of Environmental Justice (2007); Robert D. Bullard, Paul Mohai, Robin Saha, and Beverly Wright, *Toxic Wastes and Race at Twenty, 1987–2007, A Report Prepared for the United Church of Christ Justice & Witness Ministries* (2007); Robert D. Bullard and Beverly Wright, *The Wrong Complexion for Protection: How the Government Response to Disaster Endangers African American Communities* (2012).

It is too early to write the full history of health and medical care for blacks in post–Katrina New Orleans and other recent post-disaster settings. However, sources for the start of this history include: Evangeline (Vangy) Franklin, "A New Kind of Medical Disaster in the United States," in *There Is No Such Thing as a Natural Disaster: Race, Class, and Hurricane Katrina*, ed. by Chester Hartman and Gregory D. Squires (2006), 185–95; Myra A. Kleinpeter, "Rebuilding New Orleans and the Gulf Coast—Lessons Learned to Strengthen Nation's Healthcare—Response to Ferdinand's 'Public Health and Hurricane Katrina,'" *Journal of the National Medical Association* 98 (2006): 814–16; Roxanne Nelson, "Adding Insult to Injury: Five Years after Katrina," *American Journal of Nursing* 110 (2010): 19–21; Pharissa Robinson and Lila Arnaud, "Health Outcomes in Post-Katrina New Orleans: Place and Race Matter," in *State of Black New Orleans—10 Years Post Katrina*, Urban League of Greater New Orleans (2015); and Karen B. DeSalvo, "New Orleans Rises Anew: Community Health after Katrina," *Annals of Internal Medicine* 164 (2016): 57–58.

Chronology

1619—A Dutch ship brings twenty African slaves to Jamestown, Virginia, signifying the start of slavery throughout the New World. African, European, and Native American folk health practices take root across the colonies, populations, and generations.

1788—James Durham (b. 1762) is one of the nation's earliest black physicians invited to Philadelphia. He meets prominent physician Benjamin Rush, a Founding Father and signer of the Declaration of Independence.

1793—Yellow fever epidemic strikes Philadelphia. Black religious leaders Richard Allen and Absalom Jones mobilize black residents to assist the city through the epidemic.

1837—James McCune Smith (1813–1865) of New York earns medical degree in Scotland (Glasgow). He is the nation's first black physician to graduate with a formal medical degree.

1847—David Jones Peck is the first black American recipient of a medical degree from a U.S. medical school (Rush Medical School, Chicago).

1862—Freedmen's Hospital built to care for slaves and freed people during the Civil War. Affiliated with Howard University Medical School, it becomes a major resource for the national black medical profession.

1864—Rebecca Lee is the first black American woman to graduate from a U.S. medical school (New England Female Medical College, Boston).

1868—Howard University Medical Department opens. It is the first of fourteen black medical schools founded between 1868 and 1900.

1869—Robert Tanner Freeman (1856–1873) is the first black American to obtain a dental degree (Harvard Dental School).

1876—Meharry Medical College is established in Nashville, Tennessee. This institution becomes a vital avenue for the education of black doctors.

1882—Leonard Medical School, a black institution, of Shaw University is founded in Raleigh, North Carolina.

1889—Dillard University Nursing School is established in New Orleans as part of Flint Medical College. This school is the nation's oldest continuously operating black nursing school.

1890—Ida Gray Nelson Rollins (1867–1953) is the first black woman to obtain a doctor of dental surgery degree in the United States (University of Michigan).

1891—Surgeon Daniel Hale Williams organizes the nation's first black hospital: Provident Hospital and Training School for Nurses (Chicago).

1892—The *Medical and Surgical Observer* (Jackson, Tennessee) is the nation's first black medical journal published. It is edited by prominent black physician and medical educator Miles Vandahurst Link.

1893—Daniel Hale Williams performs the first successful operation involving repairing the lining of the human heart.

1895—The National Medical Association (NMA) is established in Atlanta.

1906—An Atlanta University conference on Negro problems focuses on black American health. Du Bois edits the proceedings, *The Health and Physique of the Negro American* (Atlanta University, 1906), a vital resource for later academic and public investigations.

1908—The National Association of Colored Graduate Nurses (NACGN) is founded at St. Mark's Methodist Church in New York City.

1909—The *Journal of the National Medical Association* begins publication.

1913—Daniel Hale Williams becomes the first African American member, as well as a charter member, of the American College of Surgeons.

1915—National Negro Health Week is founded at Tuskegee Institute based on the ideas of Booker T. Washington.

1923—Howard University Medical School and Meharry Medical College become the primary institutions for the education of black doctors following the closure of several black medical schools.

1923—The National Hospital Association is organized, focusing on improving the quality of black hospitals.

1932—The National Dental Association is founded. It had its roots in the Washington Society of Colored Dentists in the District of Columbia, established in 1900. Subsequently multistate black dental organizations emerged, then the NDA.

1932—The Tuskegee Study of Untreated Syphilis in the Negro Male, administered by the U.S. Public Health Service, begins in Macon County, Alabama.

1939—The National Medical Association endorses the Wagner-Dingell Bill to establish national health insurance under the Social Security Act.

1940—The National Medical Association begins meeting with the U.S. Army and Navy to urge the armed services to admit black physicians. Three hundred black physicians were called into the service in 1941.

1941—Charles R. Drew becomes the first director of the American Red Cross's Blood Bank.

1946—Congress passes the Hill-Burton law, providing funds for hospitals and other medical care facilities to expand and modernize.

1951—The National Association of Colored Graduate Nurses merges with the American Nurses Association.

1957—The Imhotep National Conference on Hospital Integration is organized by Dr. William Montague Cobb, along with the NAACP, NMA, and the Medico-Chirurgical Society of the District of Columbia.

1963—*Simkins v. Moses H. Cone Memorial Hospital.* George Simkins Jr., a black dentist and NAACP leader in Greensboro, North Carolina, assisted by the NAACP and local medical organizations, sues Moses H. Cone Memorial Hospital and other Greensboro hospitals for unlawful discrimination. The U.S. Court of Appeals Fourth Circuit rules that hospitals receiving federal funds could not set up "separate but equal" policies for black patients and black staff.

1964—The Medical Committee for Human Rights is founded. A group of predominantly white physicians, the organization teamed with other health professionals to support civil rights activities in the South. Activities grew to include protests against the AMA and other bodies to end racial discrimination policies and practices.

1964—President Lyndon B. Johnson initiates a national War on Poverty. The president spearheads federal legislation and massive social programs to reduce poverty especially linked to poor health, childhood poverty, and inadequate education.

1965—Title VI of the Civil Rights Act prohibits hospitals from receiving federal funds for racially discriminatory practices.

1965—Medicaid and Medicare legislation passes. They provide healthcare coverage to large segments of low-income citizens as well as to most all of the nation's elderly.

1966—The Charles R. Drew Post-Graduate Medical School opens in Los Angeles. The school was formed largely in response to the 1965 Watts (Los Angeles) race riot.

1966—An estimated four hundred physicians with the Medical Committee for Human Rights, the National Medical Association, and the NAACP demonstrate at the annual convention of the AMA.

1969—The Charleston (South Carolina) hospital workers strike begins. The stoppage lasts 113 days and attracts the support of Mrs. Coretta Scott King and national civil rights organizations, including SCLC (the Southern Christian Leadership Conference).

1972—The first news articles criticizing the Tuskegee Syphilis Study appear. The government ceases the study. One year later, after congressional hearings, the U.S. government settles a suit and initiates the Tuskegee Health

Benefit Program, meant to provide medical coverage and burial services for all surviving participants of the project.

1978—The *Regents of the University of California v. Bakke* case is decided.

1985—The U.S. Department of Health and Human Services and the World Health Organization (WHO) host the First International AIDS Conference in Atlanta.

1985—The first black AIDS organization is founded: Blacks Educating Blacks About Sexual Health Issues, or Babashi. Located in Philadelphia, it provided neighborhood outreach support.

1985—The report of the Secretary's Task Force on Black and Minority Health, also known as the Heckler Report, is published. One year later, among the DHHS responses to the report, it opens the Office of Minority Health.

1987—The Black Leadership Commission on AIDS is founded in New York, eventually linking over 750 churches and 1,500 AIDS-related organizations in partnership with the Centers for Disease Control and Prevention.

1988—In his bid for the Democratic Party presidential nomination, the Reverend Jesse Jackson campaigns for a national health insurance plan.

1989—Louis W. Sullivan, M.D., is appointed the head of the Department of Health and Human Services by President George H. W. Bush. In addition to secretary of HHS, Sullivan was the founding dean (in 1975) and president of the Morehouse School of Medicine for nearly two decades.

1989—Famed dancer and choreographer Alvin Ailey dies of AIDS.

1989—The Balm in Gilead organization is founded by public health activist Pernessa C. Seele. She also organizes the following church initiatives: the Black Church Week of Prayer for the Healing of AIDS, and the National Week of Prayer for the Healing of AIDS Today.

1993—AIDS becomes the leading cause of death for black American men between the ages of twenty-five and forty-four, and the second leading cause of death for black American women in this same age group.

1993—Minnie Joycelyn Elders, M.D., is appointed the nation's first black Surgeon General of the United States. She is also only the second woman to hold that position.

1994—Documentary filmmaker and AIDS activist Marlon Riggs dies at the age of thirty-seven.

1994—Executive Order 12898 on environmental justice—*Federal Actions to Address Environmental Justice in Minority Populations and Low-Income Populations*—is signed by President William J. Clinton.

1997—President William J. Clinton issues an official apology for the Tuskegee Study of Untreated Syphilis in the Negro Male, U.S. Public Health Service.

1998—David Satcher, M.D., is appointed the Surgeon General of the United States.

2005—August 29–31. Hurricane Katrina devastates New Orleans and the Gulf Coast region, including the city's healthcare system.

2010—The Patient Protection and Affordable Care Act—popularly called Obamacare—passes Congress and is signed into law. It implements a set of health insurance reforms, including the expansion of Medicaid, which enables millions of low- and middle-income citizens to obtain healthcare insurance and services.

2014—Public commemorations for Executive Order 12898 are held on the twentieth anniversary of President William J. Clinton's signing of the order on environmental justice, *Federal Actions to Address Environmental Justice in Minority Populations and Low-Income Populations*.

2017—The Meharry Medical College's Alumni Association presents a $1 million donation to the college at its 142nd commencement. Earvin "Magic" Johnson and his wife, Cookie Johnson, receive the *Ebony* Power 100 Luminary award for their worldwide support of HIV/AIDS awareness, community development for the disadvantaged, and other humanitarian causes.

Documents

HARRIET TUBMAN OBITUARY (1913)

Harriet Tubman (1822–1913) was the pivotal figure of the Underground Railroad—the secretive network in the antebellum North that assisted thousands of fugitive slaves to freedom. After the Civil War, Tubman became a cultural icon who exemplified a caregiving social leader in black American communities. Like the prominent doctors, nurses, and other health workers throughout black history, Tubman blended healing skills—in her case, nursing—with her social activism on behalf of the black American's larger struggle for freedom and equality. After her passing, Tubman's life was recounted in many obituaries and memorials written about her. Below is an excerpt from such an item that appeared in the Auburn Citizen *newspaper in Harriet's hometown in New York. In this piece, the reporter notes Tubman's nursing and folk medicine activities.*

"Memoriam: Harriet Tubman Is Dead"

"Harriet Tubman Davis, Aunt Harriet, died last night of pneumonia at the home she founded on South Street Road near here. Born lowly, she lived a life of exalted self-sacrifice and her end closes a career that has taken its place in American history. Her true services to the black race were never known but her true worth could never have been rewarded by human agency.

"It must be said that Harriet Tubman was probably the only woman who served through the war as scout, army nurse, and spy, taking her life in her hands many times in the last capacity. She was proud of the fact that she had worn 'pants' and carried a musket, canteen and haversack, accouterments which she retained after the war and left as precious relics to her colored admirers. When the war broke out she did not wait for the Emancipation

165

Proclamation but began at once forcible to free slaves. In 1863, when it was decided to use Negro troops, Harriet was instantly alert to become a nurse for a regiment. [Eventually] she was turned loose as escaped 'contraband' to browse around in the enemy's lines, only to reappear soon with valuable news of the Confederate movements.

"Harriet went to Fort Wagner after that famous charge was made there and aided in burying the black soldiers and their White officers, and in nursing the injured. Her success as a nurse, especially her ability to cure men of dysentery by means of native herbs, became so well known to the army surgeons that she was transferred by the War Department to Fernandina, Fla. which in 1863–65 was a military base, as in the Spanish-American War of 1898."

(N.A., "Memoriam: Harriet Tubman is Dead," *Auburn Citizen*, Tuesday, March 11, 1913; accessed on October 31, 2016 at http://www.harriettubman. com/memoriam2.html.)

ATLANTA UNIVERSITY CONFERENCE ON NEGRO HEALTH (1906)

Starting in 1897, Atlanta University began hosting a national conference on "Negro problems." These meetings would bring together leaders in education, health, economics, and social aid to report on these issues in various locales and regions throughout the nation. The scholar and activist W. E. B. Du Bois became the chief organizers of these conferences that gained national attention. The Atlanta Conferences also influenced government and philanthropy to increase resources for black education, social welfare, and health, especially throughout the South. The excerpt below offers a snapshot of the state of black healthcare institutions in 1906.

Hospitals

"Hospitals and careful nursing are sorely needed by Negroes. As a little North Carolina hospital reports: The hospital there has 'had a wonderful effect on the death rate among our people during the last decade. The deaths used to be three to one when compared with the whites, while the colored population was only about one-half as large as the white population. But since we have had the trained nurse, there is a marked change.'

"In the North, Negroes are admitted to the general hospitals; in the South they have separate wards or distinct institutions; outside the public hospitals which receive colored patients there are the following private hospitals of which this Conference has knowledge:

Alabama	Harris Sanatorium, Mobile; Colored Infirmary, Eufaula; Hospital, Birmingham; Hospital, Tuskegee
Arkansas	Colored Sanatorium, Little Rock
District of Columbia	Freedman's Hospital, Washington
Florida	Bruster Hospital, Faxville
Georgia	Georgia Infirmary, Savannah; Charity Hospital, Savannah; McVickar, Spelman Seminary, Atlanta; Lamar Hospital, Augusta; Burrus Sanitorium, Augusta
Indiana	Colored Hospital, care of Dr. Dupee, Evansville
Illinois	Provident Hospital, Chicago
Kansas	Douglass Hospital, Kansas City; Mitchell Hospital, Leavenworth
Kentucky	Red Cross Hospital, Covington; Citizens' National Hospital, Louisville; Louisville National Medical College
Missouri	Provident Hospital, St. Louis
Maryland	Provident Hospital, Baltimore
Mississippi	Tougaloo University Hospital, Tougaloo
North Carolina	Pinehurst Infirmary, Pinehurst; Lincoln Hospital, Durham; St. Agnes Hospital, Raleigh; State's Hospital, Winston; Good Samaritan Hospital, Charlotte; Shaw University, Raleigh
New York	Colored Home and Hospital, New York
Ohio	Colored Hospital, Cincinnati; Colley's Hospital, Cincinnati
Pennsylvania	Douglass Hospital, Philadelphia; Mercy Hospital, Philadelphia
South Carolina	Nurse Training School, Charleston
Tennessee	Hairston Infirmary, Memphis; Mercy Hospital, Nashville; Dr. J. T. Wilson's Infirmary, Nashville; The Clinic, Memphis
Texas	Colored Hospital, Dallas
Virginia	Richmond Hospital, Richmond; Women's Central League Hospital, Richmond

"Many of these hospitals have interesting histories: The Colored Hospital and Home of New York was founded by a relative of John Jay and went through the draft riots. The Freedman's Hospital grew out of the war. The Provident Hospital is one of the best organized and most efficient in the country. It has easily solved the color question, admitting both white and colored patients and employing white and colored physicians. Other institutions have been less successful. The Colored Hospital and Home of New York will not allow Negro physicians to practice in it, nor will the McVickar Hospital of Atlanta allow them to operate, although it is part of a great missionary school for Negroes."

(W. E. B. [William Edward Burghardt] Du Bois, *The Health and Physique of the Negro American: Report of a Social Study Made under the Direction of Atlanta University: Together with the Proceedings of the Eleventh Conference for the Study of the Negro Problems, Held at Atlanta University, on May the 29th, 1906* (Atlanta: Atlanta University Press, 1906), 93–95.)

JOURNAL OF THE NATIONAL MEDICAL ASSOCIATION, 1919 EDITORIAL ON BLACK HEALTH

The Journal of the National Medical Association *has been the official organ of the black physician community's National Medical Association since the organization's early founding years. First published in 1909, the JNMA has viewed medical and clinical developments in connection with the broader social conditions facing the black American population. In the editorial below published during World War I, the journal editors point out that military authorities discovered black troops were healthier in several respects compared to whites. The editors emphasize further that improved social conditions and health education for blacks in cities would also reduce the risk of social diseases in the cities—diseases that threatened both blacks and whites alike.*

Editorial: "Negro Health"

"Every Negro should be proud of the wonderful physical record our troops have made in the world war, to say nothing of their many, heroic feats. When we remember colored men were drafted, as were white men, from all walks of life, from every section of our country: and then read in the report of two eminent white authorities that our troops have more stable nerves, better eyes, are only one half as much alcoholic, and are constitutionally better physiological machines, these things should impel us to strive for an even higher record of health for our civilian population. Let us as physicians and laymen, work together to wipe out our high percentage of venereal infection. One of the best avenues of approach to this, is through a campaign of education. Our masses must be enlightened as to the seriousness of all forms of venereal diseases. There must be a campaign inaugurated and pushed, by the leaders of both races, against segregating the colored population to the worst sanitary location in the city. It is to the best interest of the municipality to make it possible by law and enforcement that all its citizens have the best environments under which to live and be healthy. If for no other reason, the city authorities should from the selfish 'self defense' viewpoint, see to it that colored people everywhere have the same opportunity for health as other people."

(Editorial, "Negro Health," *Journal of the National Medical Association*, vol. 11, n. 3 [1919]: 107–8.)

JULIUS ROSENWALD FUND'S
PROGRAM ON NEGRO HEALTH (1936)

The Julius Rosenwald Fund was established in 1917. During its early phase, it became a major philanthropic organization for social and education programs in black communities. In its first ten years, the Fund concentrated on building schoolhouses for blacks throughout the South. The next decade it broadened its operation into education and civic welfare. The Fund conducted activities involving expansion of libraries, social surveys, medical economics, and rural education. Below is an excerpt on its work to improve black health. It is from a report the Fund issued that described these two decades of the philanthropic activities.

Negro Health

"The general strategy of the Negro health program as conducted since 1928 includes:

1. Enlisting the facilities and prestige of the United States Public Health Service (through a member of its staff designated as the Fund's consultant in Negro health) to arouse and extend the interest of southern health departments and other agencies in Negro health needs and in practical steps toward meeting them; also enlisting other important national agencies such as the National Tuberculosis Association and the National Organization for Public Health Nursing to supplement the Public Health Service.
2. Aid in developing a limited number of hospitals for Negroes, conducted as demonstrations of high standards and as training centers for Negro physicians, nurses, and administrators.
3. Encouraging the use in health departments and voluntary agencies of Negro physicians and nurses, particularly public health nurses, and assisting in establishing satisfactory training for them.

4. Developing practicable methods of health education for school teachers, school children, and communities, according to policies and levels
of expense suited to southern conditions.

"The greatest amount of our contributions has gone into the development of
sixteen hospitals and clinics widely distributed throughout the North and the
South. The most notable single institution is Provident Hospital, Chicago,
which in direct affiliation with the University of Chicago has built up a
remarkably fine Negro medical staff and is in a position to offer post-graduate instruction and experience to physicians and health workers generally.

"The employment of Negro public health nurses has proceeded by leaps
and bounds and is now an established practice in southern counties and
northern cities. The campaigns against the great scourges of tuberculosis and
syphilis have proved that it is possible and financially feasible to control
these plagues. With the enlargement of public health appropriations which
are already apparent, campaigns against these diseases are likely to be put
into effect increasingly. In the control of contagious diseases it is especially
clear that the well-being of the whole population is dependent upon the
health of each group."

(Edwin R. Embree, president of the Julius Rosenwald Fund, *Julius Rosenwald Fund Review of Two Decades, 1917–1936* [Chicago, 1936], 36–37,
accessible online at https://archive.org/stream/juliusrosenwaldf033270mbp/
juliusrosenwaldf033270mbp_djvu.txt.)

W. M. COBB, *MEDICAL CARE AND THE
PLIGHT OF THE NEGRO*—NAACP, 1947

*Dr. William Montague Cobb (1904–1990) was a longtime Howard Univer-
sity Medical School faculty member. He was one of the nation's premier
physical anthropologists, medical academics, and public activists. Dr. Cobb
edited the* Journal of the National Medical Association *from the 1940s
through the 1970s, including articles that consistently challenged hospital
and medical care discrimination as well as biomedical racism. In the excerpt
below, Cobb describes the connection between black health equality and the
nation's global reputation.*

Excerpt

"The health plight of the Negro will be solved as the health plight of the
nation is solved. The Negro can no more view himself as a creature apart
than he can permit others to do so. In solving the total health problem Negro
physicians and community must assume a much heavier share of responsibil-

ity. To do this is strictly up to them. They have come far, they have yet far to go.

"From this brief review is completely obvious how badly the segregated social system has retarded improvement of help in the Negro. It is also only too clear, from the patterns which his medical advances, no matter how commendable, have had to take, that there is no real intention on the part of the majority to uproot the confines of the ghetto. Silent penetration with quiet demonstration of merit and need has certain limited values, but the Negro has nothing to hide in aims or objectives. The situation demands that America be informed and that she take notice and remove the entrenched and discriminatory practices in education, professional training and hospital customs which so blatantly indict us before the world, and impair the prestige of our leadership in the health organization of the United Nations."

(W. Montague Cobb, *Medical Care and the Plight of the Negro* [New York: NAACP, 1947], 34.)

NATIONAL BLACK NURSES ASSOCIATION — 1970

The National Black Nurses Association was formed in 1970 by a group of black nurses led by Dr. Lauranne Sams. Interested in broadening their professional connection to black communities nationwide, the few hundred initial members swelled to several thousand and dozens of chapters throughout the country in ensuing years. The black American press frequently carried announcements and reports about the NBNA's activities. The 1977 article below is from the Boston-area black newspaper, Bay State Banner.

"National Black Nurses Hold National Conference"

"The National Black Nurses Association held its 5th annual National Institute and Conference at the Sheraton Boston last week. The theme of the conference was 'A Heritage Remembered—A Practical Approach To Health Care Problems for Black Americans.' Some 500 people attended the conference from various states and cities throughout the country.

"When asked about the origins and objectives of the organization, Lauranne Sams, national president explained, 'the black nurses came together as an organization about five years ago, with various chapters becoming active in different cities.' Sams continued, 'that because of the uniqueness of health problems in the black community, it was felt that a special needs group such as the Black Nurses Association needed to be organized. We hope to increase knowledge of health problems to develop strategies to meet health needs and to promote collaboration among providers of health care for black Americans.'

"Sarah Myers, local chairperson for the New England branch and conference chairperson, said that 'locally we hope to become better known and involved in the health care problems of Boston's black community.'

"Debra Ross, when asked why she joined the organization and had come all the way from Chicago for the conference explained, 'I recently became a member for I believe that we must develop unity and this can be done by being in touch with other black nurses throughout the country.'"

(T. Edwards, "National Black Nurses Hold Annual Conference," *Bay State Banner* [Boston, MA], November 10, 1977: 9.)

DEPARTMENT OF HEALTH AND HUMAN SERVICES, HECKLER REPORT — 1985

In 1985, the secretary of the Department of Health and Human Services, Margaret M. Heckler, released the groundbreaking survey The Secretary's Task Force Report on Black and Minority Health, *popularly known as the Heckler Report. The report became the benchmark for federal health policy involving blacks and other racial minorities in the subsequent decades. What follows is Heckler's letter that introduces the exhaustive, multivolume report. The report itself is an abundant resource for black health history research.*

Letter from Heckler Report

"The Secretary of Health and Human Services

"Washington, DC 20201

"In January 1984—ten months after becoming Secretary of Health and Human Services—I sent *Health, United States, 1983* to the Congress. It was the annual report card on the health status of the American people.

"That report—like its predecessors—documented significant progress: Americans were living longer, infant mortality had continued to decline—the overall American health picture showed almost uniform improvement.

"But, and that 'but' signaled a sad and significant fact; *there was a continuing disparity in the burden of death and illness experienced by Blacks and other minority Americans as compared with our nation's population as a whole.*

"That disparity has existed ever since accurate federal record keeping began—more than a generation ago. And although our health charts do itemize steady gains in the health status of minority Americans, the stubborn disparity remained—an affront both to our ideals and to the ongoing genius of American medicine.

"I felt—passionately that it was time to decipher the message inherent in that disparity. In order to unravel the complex picture provided by our data and experience, I established a Secretarial Task Force whose broad assignment was the comprehensive investigation of the health problems of Blacks, Native Americans, Hispanics and Asian/Pacific Islanders.

"The Task Force . . . was further charged with finding ways for our department to exert leadership, influence and initiative to close the existing gap. The report is comprehensive. Its analysis is thoughtful. Its thrust is masterful. It sets the framework for meeting the challenge—for improving the health of minorities.

"It can—it should—mark the beginning of the end of the health disparity that has, for so long, cast a shadow on the otherwise splendid American track record of ever improving health.

"Margaret M. Heckler

"Secretary"

(U.S. Department of Health and Human Resources, [Margaret M. Heckler, Secretary of HHS], *Report of the Secretary's Task Force on Black and Minority Health* [popularly known as the *Heckler Report*], 1985.)

SURGEON GENERAL COMMENTARY, DR. JOYCELYN ELDERS—1994

Dr. Joycelyn Elders (M.D., Ph.D.) served as the surgeon general to the United States in 1993 and 1994. She was the first black American appointed to that position. Dr. Elders was a strong advocate for community-based health policies, especially public health education, as the most important means to reduce health problems linked to drug abuse, teenage pregnancy, and poverty. In her "Health Commentary" article in the NAACP's Crisis *magazine, Dr. Elders promotes her approach to curtail the black health crisis engulfing black communities at that time. She points out that high rates of unemployment and homelessness are associated with poor health. Dr. Elders then elaborates on other factors.*

Excerpt

"[E]ducation is inversely associated with mortality. In 1989–90, for men and women 24–44 years old, persons not completing high school had mortality rates three times greater than those of college graduates. For persons 45–64 years old not completing high school, the mortality rates were twice those of college graduates.

"[Also] unmarried teenage mothers often drop out of school and remain unemployed. In 1991, 68% of black mothers of newborns were unmarried, compared to 22% of white mothers. . . . Poverty among black children (46%) is almost 3 times as frequent as white children (16%).

"The health of African-Americans is also aggravated by homicide and legal intervention [i.e., prison] rates, [in addition to] poverty, infant mortality, and high mortality rates from preventable diseases. Homicide and legal intervention rates are 7 times higher among African-American males than white males. . . .

"So, even though African Americans are more likely to require health care, under our current system they are less likely to receive healthcare services. For example, fifty percent of poor African-American women with breast cancer already have metastatic disease by the time they enter the hospital, compared to nine percent of white and sixteen percent of Hispanic women. Another example is that recent studies show that people of color are far less likely to receive treatment for AIDS related pneumonia (Pneumocystis carinii pneumonia, commonly known as PCP), an illness that is largely preventable by taking inexpensive, widely available drugs. . . .

"As our nation now engages in aggressive debate over various health care reform goals and strategies, I would like to describe my priorities for improving the Nation's Health:

SURGEON GENERAL'S STRATEGY FOR CHANGE:

1. Provision of universal access to health care services for all Americans
2. Emphasis on Prevention and Primary Care
3. Comprehensive Health Education
4. Increase individual and community RESPONSIBILITY for health
5. Early Childhood Education
6. Parent Education
7. Every Child born in America a planned wanted child
8. Male Responsibility
9. School-Based Health Services
10. Hope

"Each one of us must play a strategic role if we are to succeed in improving the HEALTH (*sic*) of African Americans. We must INSIST on a health care system which guarantees ALL Americans access to health care without regard to age, gender, race or socioeconomic status. And together, we must restructure our health system to make HEALTH a priority—by focusing on prevention and health education. As your Surgeon General, I call upon you— leaders in the African American community—to join me in improving America's HEALTH through PREVENTION."

(Dr. Joycelyn Elders, "Health Commentary: The Future of Health Care for African Americans," *Crisis*, 101, 7 [October 1994]: 25, 30.)

PROCLAMATION OF BLACK
CHURCHES ON STOPPING AIDS—1994

The African American Clergy Summit on HIV took place in 1994. Also at that time, a meeting on the AIDS problem occurred between black religious leaders and the Clinton administration. Eventually black clergy leaders composed and signed A Proclamation from the Balm in Gilead *titled "The African American Clergy's Declaration of War on HIV/AIDS." Here is an excerpt of that proclamation. At this time, The Balm in Gilead was a new community-based organization founded to unite black churches to work collectively in black communities expanding education and awareness about the AIDS problem. Such proclamations became effective means to draw more churches nationwide into black faith-based programs and campaigns like the Balm in Gilead.*

Excerpt

"The African-American Church has a long and distinguished tradition of leading its people to light in times of great suffering, and of caring for its parishioners. It has a proud history of pastoral activism and has proven itself a formidable mobilizer of congregations. . . . The church's godly mission is to minister love and support to its congregations, and to forsake no one, yet, until today, it has not assumed its proper mantle of responsibility in this time of chaos caused by the ravages of AIDS to mind, body and soul of our people.

"By this proclamation, we declare our intent to do all in our power to eradicate the scourge of AIDS in our time; to wage a war on fear and ignorance of AIDS/HIV, from the pulpit and in our institutions, until such a time as AIDS is no longer a threat to the lives of the people, and we call upon our fellow clergy, men and women, to do the same.

"Therefore we vow to develop comprehensive AIDS prevention programs for our youth, [and] for and with our congregations and communities; to provide supportive counseling to Persons Living with AIDS and to their non-infected families and loved ones; and to preach consciousness-raising sermons about AIDS prevention and compassion for all, regardless of sexual orientation, drug dependency, or lifestyle choices."

(The Balm in Gilead, Inc., *The Power of Prayer: 25th Anniversary of the Week of Prayer for the Healing of AIDS*, accessible at: http://www.balmingilead.org/tbig/wp-content/uploads/2015/07/Web-version-THE-POWER-OF-PRAYER-fnl.pdf.)

BLACK CHURCHES OF NEW YORK
ANTI-AIDS PROGRAM—1996

Below is an article by Andrew Jacobs, "A New Antagonist for AIDS," that appeared in the New York Times, *December 1, 1996. It describes the growing importance during the mid-1990s of the black church in the struggle to help the victims of AIDS and increase public awareness about the disease. In the article, Ms. Pernessa C. Seele, an administrator at Harlem Hospital in New York City, explains her motivation for becoming involved in assisting the victims of AIDS.*

A New Antagonist for AIDS

"In the 1980s, as gay white men downtown waged their highly public fight against AIDS, church leaders uptown in Harlem shook their heads disapprovingly. 'Ministers up here just figured it was divine retribution for sinful behavior,' recalls Dr. Preston R. Washington, the pastor of Memorial Baptist Church on West 115th Street.

"But these days, Dr. Washington knows differently. His address book is filled with the crossed-out names of friends who have died of AIDS, and in the last few years, he has buried 20 parishioners who succumbed to the disease. While in 1986, 24 percent of those with AIDS were black nationwide, a decade later that figure has nearly doubled. These days, a black woman is 16 times as likely to contract H.I.V., the virus that causes AIDS, than a white [woman], and most children with the disease are black.

"'The church I knew in the South was always a place you could bring your pain, sickness and grief,' Ms. Seele said. 'I couldn't bear the silence anymore.'

"Ms. Seele began by approaching local members of the clergy and asking them to pray for people with AIDS. Later, she asked them to do more. Today, Ms. Seele's organization, the Balm in Gilead, works with 60 churches citywide, helping them provide AIDS education and outreach programs."

(Andrew Jacobs, "A New Antagonist for AIDS," *New York Times*, December 1, 1996.)

SURGEON GENERAL DAVID SATCHER
ON HEALTHY PEOPLE CAMPAIGN—2000

In 1998, David Satcher (M.D., Ph.D.) was appointed the surgeon general of the United States. Satcher had become a nationally prominent figure in medicine and public health focusing on black and minority American health issues. During his career, Satcher became a leader at the King-Drew Medical Center in Los Angeles, at the Charles R. Drew Postgraduate Medical School, and as the president of Meharry Medical College (1982 to 1993). What follows are his remarks at a public meeting initiating the Healthy People 2010 campaign. The Healthy People campaigns began in 1979 to improve health levels promoted by federal agencies and hundreds of membership organizations. Satcher's remarks are a clear enunciation of the health equality ideal.

Remarks by Satcher at Healthy People 2010 Campaign

"Good morning. I am delighted to be here, and I want to join Secretary Shalala, Secretary Sullivan, and Dr. Richmond in welcoming you to this historic event.

"The fact that each one of them is here on the platform today is testimony to the fact that something special is going on here today. Zora Neale Hurston said that "The present is an egg laid by the past that has the future in its shell." Today, under the watchful and nurturing eye of Dr. Shalala, Dr. Sullivan, [and] many others, we are witnessing the birth of another Healthy People that will grow and develop over the next ten years. . . .

"Healthy People 2010's two overarching goals of increasing years and quality of life and of eliminating racial and ethnic disparities in health are also indicative of our connection to the past and the major achievements we hope to see by the end of this decade. . . .

"We have heard from many people who have told us that our goal of eliminating disparities by 2010 is overly ambitious. We have responded by saying that in the 21st century, neither history nor humanity can settle for less. That commitment to eliminate disparities has already galvanized communities, states, and non-governmental organizations throughout the country to develop their own commitments and strategies. . . .

"Together, as a nation, we must move toward a balanced community health system—one that makes access to quality care available to all; that balances early detection of disease with health promotion and disease prevention; that draws on the involvement of the community, including homes, community schools, churches and other faith-based organizations, and civic and local groups."

(David Satcher, M.D., Ph.D., "Opening Remarks Healthy People 2010 Launch," Assistant Secretary for Health and Surgeon General, Office of Public Health and Science, Washington, DC, January 25, 2000; accessible online at http://www.surgeongeneral.gov/about/previous/satcher/speeches/healthy1.html.)

Notes

INTRODUCTION

1. John Hope Franklin, *The Color Line: Legacy for the Twenty-First Century* (Columbia: University of Missouri Press, 1994), n.p.; accessed August 20, 2015 at http://jhfc.duke.edu/johnhopefranklin/quotes.html.

1. SLAVERY AND THE MEDICAL ROOTS

1. Excerpt from Frances Ann Kemble, *Journal of a Residence on a Georgia Plantation in 1838–1839*, ed. by John A. Scott (New York: Alfred A. Knopf), 224–41; reprinted in *Black Women in White America: A Documentary History*, ed. by Gerda Lerner (New York: Vintage, 1973), 49.
2. W. E. B. Du Bois, *The Souls of Black Folk* (1903), n.p.; accessed October 20, 2015, online at http://www.gutenberg.org/files/408/408-h/408-h.htm.
3. Theodore D. Weld, *American Slavery As It Is: Testimony of a Thousand Witnesses* (1839), 45; accessed June 20, 2017 at: http://docsouth.unc.edu/neh/weld/weld.html.
4. Ibid., 47.
5. Ibid.

2. BATTLING FOR LIFE IN THE CIVIL WAR AND NADIR ERAS

1. W. Montague Cobb, "A Short History of the Freedmen's Hospital," *Journal of the National Medical Association* 54, no. 3 (1962), 277.
2. Charles B. Purvis, quoted by Cobb, ibid., 277.
3. Rev. William J. Simmons, *Men of Mark: Eminent, Progressive and Rising* (Cleveland: 1887), 692.
4. Cobb, "A Short History," 275–76. Over the years, Freedmen's Hospital leadership cited this heritage time and again in their many future struggles to win government aid and public

support for the institution. In 1961, President John F. Kennedy signed a law transferring Freedmen's to Howard University, with plans and funding to immensely increase its buildings and programs.

5. C. C. Penick, "The Colored Race as a Problem in Sanitation," in Kentucky State Board of Health, *Proceedings, Addresses, and Discussions of a Public Health Conference, Held at Louisville, Kentucky, May 24 and 25, 1887*, 134–5; quote of G. B. Thornton, M.D., president, Memphis Board of Health, "Negro Mortality," ibid., 135.

6. John Blassingame, *Black New Orleans, 1860–1880* (Chicago: University of Chicago Press, 1973), 163–64, quote on 164.

7. Frederick L. Hoffman, *Race Traits and Tendencies of the American Negro* (New York: Macmillan, 1896), 95, 329.

8. Murrell, cited in David McBride, *From TB to AIDS: Epidemics among Urban Blacks since 1900* (Albany, NY: SUNY Press, 1991),18–20.

9. W. E. B. Du Bois (ed.), *The Health and Physique of the Negro American: Report of a Social Study Made under the Direction of Atlanta University . . . May the 29th, 1906* (Atlanta: Atlanta University Press, 1906), 104.

10. United States National Library of Medicine, *Changing the Face of Medicine—Dr. Rebecca J. Cole*, accessed at https://www.nlm.nih.gov/changingthefaceofmedicine/physicians/biography_66.html.

11. Du Bois, *Health and Physique*, 96, 106.

12. Ibid., 110.

13. La Vinia Delois Jennings (ed.), *Zora Neale Hurston, Haiti, and* Their Eyes Were Watching God (Evanston, IL: Northwestern University Press, 2013), Hurston quote on 198.

14. Anna de Costa Banks, "The Work of a Small Hospital and Training School in the South," *Eighth Annual Report of the Hampton Training School for Nurses and Dixie Hospital* (Hampton, Virginia, 1898–1899), 23–38, reprinted in *Black Women in the Nursing Profession: A Documentary History*, ed. by Darlene C. Hine (New York: Garland, 1985), 5 includes quote.

3. THE BLACK MEDICAL WORLD

1. "An Address on the History of the National Medical Association, T. A. Walker [Baton Rouge, La.], NMA-Philadelphia, August 22, 1906," in John A. Kenney, "Some Notes on the History of the National Medical Association," *Journal of the National Medical Association* (*JNMA*) 25 (1933): 98.

2. John A. Kenney, "Health Problems of the Negroes," *The Annals of the American Academy of Political and Social Science* 37 (1911): 110.

3. Ibid., 112–13; Boyd quote on p. 113.

4. Booker T. Washington, "Training Colored Nurses at Tuskegee," *The American Journal of Nursing* 11 (1910): 168.

5. John A. Kenney, "Some Facts Concerning Negro Nurse Training Schools and Their Graduates," *JNMA* 11 (1919): 54.

6. Dorothy Deming, "The Negro Nurse in Public Health," *Opportunity: Journal of Negro Life* 15 (November 1937), 333–35; reprinted in *Black Women in the Nursing Profession: A Documentary History*, ed. by Darlene C. Hine (New York: Garland, 1985), 98.

7. Ibid., 98, 99.

8. Henry R. M. Landis, "The Negro Nurse in Public Health Work," *Child Health Bulletin* 3, no. 1 (1927): 20.

9. E. H. Beardsley, *A History of Neglect: Health Care for Blacks and Mill Workers in the Twentieth-Century South* (Knoxville: University of Tennessee Press, 1987), 37.

10. Brian Dolinar (ed.), *The Negro in Illinois: The WPA Papers* (Urbana: University of Illinois Press, 2013), 153, quote is of WPA writer.

11. H. M. Green, M.D., Ph.D., "A Brief Study of the Hospital Situation among Negroes," *JNMA* 22 (1930): 112.

12. [Letter from a Woman Migrant], ca. May–June, 1917; No. 71, in *African Americans in the Industrial Age: A Documentary History, 1915–1945*, ed. by Joe W. Trotter and Earl Lewis (Boston: Northeastern University Press, 1996), 99.

13. Beardsley, *History of Neglect*, 156–86.

4. CIVIL RIGHTS, HEALTH RIGHTS

1. Gunnar Myrdal, *An American Dilemma: The Negro Problem and Modern Democracy* (New York: Harper & Row, 1944; 1962), 927.

2. Thomas F. Pettigrew, *A Profile of the Negro American* (New York: D. Van Nostrand, 1964), 78–80; Abram Kardiner and Lionel Ovesey, *The Mark of Oppression: A Psychosocial Study of the American Negro* (New York: Norton, 1951), 343.

3. See Charles S. Johnson, *The Negro College Graduate* (1938); and Monroe N. Work, *Negro Year Book: An Annual Encyclopedia of the Negro, 1931–1932* (1931) and *1937–1938* (1937). Quote is from Myrdal, *An American Dilemma*, 324–25.

4. James Summerville, *Educating Black Doctors: A History of Meharry Medical College* (Tuscaloosa: University of Alabama Press, 2002), 93.

5. Wilkie quote in Myrdal, *An American Dilemma*, 1008–9.

6. Roy Wilkins, "Nurses Go to War," *Crisis* (February 1943), 42–44; quote on 42.

7. Roosevelt Institute, "FDR's Second Bill of Rights: 'Necessitous Men Are Not Free Men,'" (January 11, 1944); accessed July 20, 2017 at http://rooseveltinstitute.org/fdrs-second-bill-rights-necessitous-men-are-not-free-men/.

8. Herbert M. Morais, *The History of the Negro in Medicine* (New York: Publishers Company/Association for the Study of Negro Life and History, 1968), 148, includes quote; see also Quentin Young, "The Urban Hospital: Inequity, High Tech, and Low Performance," in *Reforming Medicine: Lessons of the Last Quarter Century*, ed. by Victor W. Sidel and Ruth Sidel (New York: Pantheon, 1984), 33–49.

9. Detroit Commission on Community Relations, *Medical and Hospital Study Committee Report* (1956), 24; quoted in David McBride, *From TB to AIDS: Epidemics among Urban Blacks since 1900* (Albany, NY: SUNY Press, 1991), 148.

10. James P. Comer, *Beyond Black and White* (New York: Quadrangle Books, 1972), 39.

11. W. Montague Cobb, *Seventh Imhotep National Conference on Hospital Integration*, May 1963; quoted in Morais, *The Negro in Medicine*, 159.

12. Max Seham, "Discrimination against Negroes in Hospitals," *New England Journal of Medicine* 271 (October 29, 1964): 940–43.

5. WAR ON POVERTY AND THE "MEDICAL GHETTO"

1. Amanda Moore, "Tracking Down Martin Luther King Jr.'s Words on Health Care," *Huffpost*, January 18, 2013; accessed June 17, 2017 at http://www.huffingtonpost.com/amanda-moore/martin-luther-king-health-care_b_2506393.html.

2. Martin Luther King Jr. [unidentified speech], March 4, 1968; cited by National Archives, *JFK Assassination Records*, accessed June 16, 2017 at https://www.archives.gov/research/jfk/select-committee-report/part-2-king-findings.html.

3. John L. S. Holloman Jr., "Future Role of the Ghetto Physician," in *Medicine in the Ghetto*, ed. by John C. Norman (New York: Appleton-Century-Crofts, 1969), 133–52; quotes on 150, 134.

4. Health PAC, *The American Health Empire: Power, Profits, and Politics* (New York: Vintage, 1971), 214.

5. James H. Carter, "Psychiatry, Racism and Aging," *Journal of the American Geriatrics Society* 20 (1972): 343–46; James H. Carter, "Psychiatry's Insensitivity to Racism and Aging," *Psychiatric Opinion* 10 (1973): 21–25, quote on 21.

6. William H. Grier and Price M. Cobbs, *Black Rage* (New York: Bantam Books, 1969), quoted by J. M. Metzl, *The Protest Psychosis: How Schizophrenia Became a Black Disease* (Boston: Beacon, 2009), 124.

7. James P. Comer, *Beyond Black and White* (New York: Quadrangle Books, 1972), 117.

8. Carl C. Bell, *The Sanity of Survival: Reflections on Community Mental Health and Wellness* (Chicago: Third World Press, 2004), xxiii.

9. Martin Luther King, Jr. [unidentified speech], March 4, 1968; cited by National Archives, *JFK Assassination Records*, accessed June 16, 2017 at https://www.archives.gov/research/jfk/select-committee-report/part-2-king-findings.html.

10. *Oral History Interview with Mary Moultrie* [Typescript, 29 pp.], Int. by Jean-Claude Bouffard, July 28, 1982, *Avery Research Center at the College of Charleston, S.C.*, 4.

11. James T. Wooten, "14 Rights Leaders Support Strikers," *New York Times*, April 21, 1969.

12. Wooten, "100 Negroes Seized in Charleston Protest March," *New York Times,* April 27, 1969; includes quote. Wooten, "Charleston Is an Armed Camp as 142 Are Held," *New York Times*, April 29, 1969.

13. Ibid.

14. A. H. Raskin, "A Union with 'Soul,'" *New York Times*, March 22, 1970.

15. "Family Planning to Get Poor's Aid: Bronx Residents Recruited for Work in Centers," *New York Times*, November 2, 1969.

16. Helen Rodriguez-Trias, "The Women's Health Movement: Women Take Power," *Reforming Medicine: Lessons of the Last Quarter Century*, ed. by Victor W. Sidel and Ruth Sidel (New York: Pantheon, 1984), 110.

17. Joseph D. Beasley, "View from Louisiana," *Family Planning Perspectives* 1, No. 1 (1969): 15. Beasley (M.D.) was the director of the Center for Population and Family Studies at Tulane University School of Medicine and of the Louisiana Family Planning Program. He also held national positions as chair of the National Advisory Council of the Center for Family Planning Program Development, as well as the chair of the Executive Committee of Planned Parenthood-World Population (ibid., 2). For a case study of a neighborhood center in Detroit in which black women resisted the criticism of local black nationalists that birth control was a form of genocide, see Nancy Milio, *9226 Kercheval: The Storefront That Did Not Burn* (Ann Arbor: University of Michigan Press, 1970).

18. U.S. Department of Health, Education, and Welfare, *Final Report of the Tuskegee Syphilis Study Ad Hoc Advisory Panel, U.S. Department of Health, Education and Welfare, 1973*, 14.

19. Ibid., 18.

20. *Richard Nixon, President of the United States: 1969–1974, 155-Statement on Signing the National Sickle Cell Anemia Control Act, May 16, 1972*; accessed online June 18, 2017 at http://www.presidency.ucsb.edu/ws/?pid=3413.

6. CONFRONTING THE BLACK HEALTH CRISIS

1. J. Alfred Cannon, "Re-Africanization: The Last Alternative for Black America," *Phylon* 38 (1977), 203 (emphasis added).

2. E. Richard Brown, "Medicare and Medicaid: Band-Aids for the Old and Poor," in *Reforming Medicine: Lessons for the Last Quarter Century*, ed. by Victor W. Sidel and Ruth Sidel (New York: Pantheon, 1984), 65.

3. Harold Washington, "Barriers to Black Physicians and Health Care," *JNMA* 76 (1984): 12.

4. Joyce A. Ladner and Ruby M. Gourdine, "Adolescent Pregnancy in the African-American Community," in *Black Health Issues in the Black Community*, ed. by Ronald L. Braithwaite and Sandra E. Taylor (San Francisco: Jossey-Bass, 1992), 206.

5. Edward H. Beardsley, *A History of Neglect: Health Care for Blacks and Mill Workers in the Twentieth-Century South* (Knoxville: University of Tennessee Press, 1987), 274.

6. Dorothy K. Newman et al., *Protest, Politics, and Prosperity: Black Americans and White Institutions, 1940–1975* (New York: Pantheon, 1978), 190; Byllye Y. Avery, "The Health Status of Black Women," in *Black Health Issues in the Black Community*, ed. by Braithwaite and Taylor, 40.

7. M. Alfred Haynes M.D., "Charles R. Drew Postgraduate Medical School," *The Western Journal of Medicine* 140 (1984): 308–319.

8. Margaret Heckler, [Letter introducing], United States Department of Health and Human Services, *Report of the Secretary's Task Force on Black and Minority Health* (1985).

9. Bernard Weinraub, "Jackson Calls for a National Health Care Plan," *New York Times*, June 23, 1988.

10. Muriel L. Whetstone, "New AIDS Scare for Heterosexuals: The Increasing Threat to Black Women," *Ebony* (April 1994), 118–20; quote on 119 includes remark by Denise K.

11. Frederick G. Murray and Joycelyn M. Elders, "Diabetes and the Black Community," in *Black Health Issues in the Black Community*, ed. by Braithwaite and Taylor, 129.

7. THE AIDS ERA AND THE TIME OF KATRINA

1. D. Mendell and D. Little, "Poverty, Crime Still Stalk City's Middle-Class Blacks," *Chicago Tribune*, July 27, 2003.

2. Louis Sullivan, quoted by Mary-Christine Phillip, "AIDS: Fighting a Killer through Education: Despite Heavy Toll on Hispanic and Black Men, Women, Children, Most AIDS Research Focuses on Whites," *Black Issues in Higher Education* 10 (April 8, 1993): 23.

3. UPI, "The City's public health commissioner, reacting to the refusal...,"*UPI NewsTrack*, February 7, 1986; accessed online October 16, 2016 at http://infoweb.newsbank.com.ezaccess.libraries.psu.edu/resources/doc/nb/news/15698D4DEED85AF8?p=AWNB. See also Steve Gorman, "School officials in the nation's capital barred a student . . . ," *UPI NewsTrack*, September 5, 1985; Martha E. Stern (ed.), *Health Care Crisis: We Can Make a Difference! A National Conference on Alleviating Health Care Problems in Minority and Poor Communities, Conference Proceeding November 15 and 16, 1985, Howard University* (Washington, DC: Government of the District of Columbia/UDHHS, [1985]).

4. D. L. Kirp and R. Bayer, "Needles and Race," *Atlantic* 272 (July 1993): 38–42; comment by Reverend Graylan Ellis-Hagler on 39.

5. *About the Balm in Gilead*, www.balmingilead.org, retrieved August 13, 2003; "Welcome: A Message from Pernessa C. Seele," ibid., includes quote.

6. "Black Clergy Gather to Fight AIDS," *Christian Century* 110 (October 20, 1993): 1009.

7. P. C. Seele, "Creating Positive Change with the Power of Prayer," *About . . . Time* (Rochester, NY: January–February 1999), 36; includes quote by Jakes.

8. *SisterLove, Inc.* Webpage accessed August 2, 2016 at http://www.sisterlove.org/about-us/.

9. Mike Farley, "Health Care Debate Rages On," *Black Enterprise* 22 (May 1992), quote of Louis Stokes is on p. 20.

10. Gary C. Dennis, M.D., "Creating Great Leaders in Health Care, with a Vision for the New Millennium," *JNMA* 90 (1998): 520.

11. Tracy M. Walton Jr., M.D., "Health-Care Reform: The National Medical Association's Number One Priority," *JNMA* 86 (1994): 735–36; quote on 735.

12. Ibid.

13. Kevin Sack, "Epidemic Takes Toll on Black Women," *New York Times*, July 3, 2001, includes quotes.

14. T. C. Quinn, "Commentary on the 4th Conference on Retroviruses and Opportunistic Infections," *The Hopkins HIV Report*, March 1997, accessed May 21, 2018 at: http://www.thebody.com/content/art42892.html, includes quote by D. Ho.

15. Sheryl Gay Stolberg, "Epidemic of Silence: A Special Report: Eyes Shut, Black America Is Being Ravaged by AIDS," *New York Times*, June 29, 1998.

16. Lance Hill, "Poverty Skyrockets in New Orleans," *Louisiana Weekly*, October 24, 2011, accessed October 15, 2016, at http://www.louisianaweekly.com/poverty-skyrockets-in-new-orleans/.

Index

King, Coretta Scott, 101–104, 102
King, Martin Luther, Jr., 87, 90
Knights and Daughters of Tabor, 67–68
Koop, C. Everett, 129

lactose intolerance, 3
Landis, Henry, Dr., 48
Latino Americans, xii, 95, 152
lead poisoning, 140, 144
Lear, Walter J., 81
life expectancy, 64, 88

Mahoney, Marie Eliza, 32
malaria, 24
male suffrage, 17
malnutrition, 3, 90
MAP. *See* Minority AIDS Project
Martin Luther King Jr. General Hospital, 116
Mather, Cotton, 8
mayoral candidates, black, 116
MCAT. *See* Medical College Admissions Test
McBride, Andrew D., Jr., 134
McCune Smith, James, 12–14, 14
MCHR. *See* Medical Committee for Human Rights
MDR-TB. *See* multidrug resistant tuberculosis
measles, 64
Medicaid, 90–91, 98, 109, 111, 143; ACA and, 152; AIDS and, 147; blocking funding for, 113; eligibility for, 113; flaws of, 114; patient treatment on, 114
medical care gaps, 112
medical care network, 118; all-black, 65
medical care system: national, 109; national spending in, 119
Medical College Admissions Test (MCAT), 117
Medical Committee for Civil Rights, 82
Medical Committee for Human Rights (MCHR), 81, 82
medical experimentation, unethical, 108
"Medical Ghetto", 87–109, 102, 108
medical schools, black, 117; development of, 30; hospitals and, 49; Morehouse Medical School, 116

Medicare, 90–91, 98, 109, 143; flaws of, 114
medicine, academic-based, xi
Meharry Medical College of Walden University, 29, 46
meningitis, 64
mental health, 64–65, 89–90, 95–96, 97; preventive care for, 125; public institutions for, 97
mental illness, 113
Mercy Hospital, 68
Mfume, Kweisi, 147
midwives, black, 31, 56, 69
migrants, 44
militancy, black, 107
military, 46
Minority AIDS Project (MAP), 137
Missing Persons: Minorities in the Health Professions, 149
Model Cities Program, 94
Morehouse Medical School, 116
mortality rates, 38, 65, 88, 113, 120; from AIDS, 135, 146; infant, 88, 116; from TB, 64, 88
Muhammad, Elijah, 135
multidrug resistant tuberculosis (MDR-TB), 127
music, 5, 149, 152; gospel, 147; rap, 124
My Life in Camp with the 33rd US Colored Troops, 14

NACGN. *See* National Association of Colored Graduate Nurses
Nadir Era, xii, 152; black life during, 17–35; health reforms during, 25–30
National Advisory Committee on Civil Disorders, 91
National Association of Colored Graduate Nurses (NACGN), 32, 39, 71
National Black Nurses Association (NBNA), 144
National Black Women's Health Project, 116
national healthcare insurance, 76, 142, 143
National Health Program (NHP), 122–123
National Hospital Association (NHA), 45, 54
National Institutes of Health, 143

National Medical Association (NMA), 28–29, 39, 143–145
National Medical Research Act of 1974, 108
National Negro Health News, 59
National Negro Health Week, 59, 97
National Organization of Public Health Nursing, 47
National Sickle Cell Anemia Control Act of 1972, 109
National Urban League (NUL), 102
National Youth Administration (NYA), 60
natural disasters, 112, 129. *See also* Hurricane Katrina
NBNA. *See* National Black Nurses Association
needle exchange program, 136
Needleman, Herbert, Dr., 140
Negro Health Bureau, 48
"Negro Health" movement, 38, 41
"Negro Hospital Renaissance", 52
Negro professional, 66
neoliberal economics, xiv, 143
neoslavery, xiii
New Activists, 109, 119, 121, 152; AIDS epidemic and, 126, 133–134, 137; "Battlers" and, 112; health leaders, 116; leaders of, 145; stepping forward as, 132
New Deal, xiii, 60, 61; initiatives, 111
New Ghetto, xiv, 112; black health crisis and, 114; drugs in, 125; emergence of, 114; escape from, 127; poverty, 117; spreading of, 132
New Negro, 45, 49
New Orleans, 152; black health disparities in, 151; black health in, 149; citizens of, 149; crime rates in, 150; drug treatment facilities in, 150; health insurance lacking in, 151; health system rebuilding in, 150; medical resources in, 149; mental health facilities in, 150; post-Katrina federal funding, 151; poverty in, 151; Veterans' Affairs Medical Center, 150. *See also* Hurricane Katrina
NHA. *See* National Hospital Association
NHP. *See* National Health Program
niacin deficiency, 3

Niagara Movement, 38
NMA. *See* National Medical Association
North Jersey Medical Society, 40
Notes on Virginia, 8
Novello, Antonia, 129
NUL. *See* National Urban League
nurses, black, 31; Army Nurse Corps, 46, 71; during interwar years, 50; NACGN, 32, 39, 71; NBNA, 144; *The Pathfinders: A History of the Progress of Colored Graduate Nurses*, 32; schools, 32–35. *See also* Provident Hospital and Training School for Nurses
nutrition, 2–3, 90, 132
NYA. *See* National Youth Administration

Obama, Barack, 151, 152
Obamacare, 152
Office of Equal Opportunity, U.S. (OEO), 94, 98
Office of Minority Health (OMH), 120
Office of Negro Health Work, 59
OMH. *See* Office of Minority Health
Onesimus, 8
ONE VOICE, 147

Parran, Thomas, Dr., 60
The Pathfinders: A History of the Progress of Colored Graduate Nurses, 32
Patient Protection and Affordable Care Act (ACA), 152
pellagra, 3
philanthropic programs, 98–99
physician workforce: small-group practices, 120; specialties in, 119; women in, 118
Plessy v. Ferguson, 21
pneumonia, 38
policies, discriminatory, xii
political equality, xiv, 87
politics: conflict in, 112; conservative, 117
pollution, 112, 129, 132
poverty, 38; black families in, 128; elimination of, xii; line, 113; in New Ghetto, 117; in New Orleans, 151; patterns of, 112; single-parent families in, 115; urban, 112; war on, xiii, 87, 87–109, 102, 108, 111